MORE
MUSCLE

Human Kinetics

Library of Congress Cataloging-in-Publication Data

Sprague, Ken.
    More muscle / Ken Sprague.
      p.   cm.
    Includes index.
    ISBN 0-87322-899-5
    1. Weight training. 2. Bodybuilding. 3. Body, Human. I. Title.
  GV546.S686 1996
  613.7' 13--dc20   96-2482
                                                          CIP

ISBN: 0-87322-899-5

Information on fat, calorie, and sodium content of foods listed in chapter 10 taken from *Code of Federal Regulations* (1995), Title 21, 101.60-62. Washington, DC: U.S. Government Printing Office.

Photographs courtesy of Sam Doane; Complete Production Services, Ltd.; Photo Design; Kipling Rock Productions; and John Bauguess.

Arnold Schwarzenegger quote on p. 12 from the film *Pumping Iron.*

Developmental Editor: Julia Anderson; **Assistant Editors:** Jacqueline Eaton Blakley and John Wentworth; **Editorial Assistant:** Coree Schutter; **Copyeditor:** Michael Ryder; **Proofreader:** Jacqueline Seebaum; **Indexer:** Barbara Cohen; **Text Design and Layout:** Bob Reuther; **Typesetting and Layout:** Ruby Zimmerman; **Cover Designer:** Jack Davis; **Cover Photograph:** Ray Malace; **Printer:** Braun-Brumfield

Printed in the United States of America   10 9 8 7 6 5 4 3 2 1

Human Kinetics
P.O. Box 5076, Champaign, IL 61825-5076
1-800-747-4457
http://www.hkusa.com

Canada: Human Kinetics, Box 24040, Windsor, ON N8Y 4Y9
1-800-465-7301 (in Canada only)
humank@hkcanada.com

Europe: Human Kinetics,
P.O. Box IW14, Leeds LS16 6TR, United Kingdom
(44) 1132 781708
humank@hkeurope.com

Australia: Human Kinetics, 2 Ingrid Street, Clapham 5062, South Australia
(08) 371 3755
humank@hkaustralia.com

New Zealand: Human Kinetics, P.O. Box 105-231, Auckland 1
(09) 523 3462
humank@hknewz.com

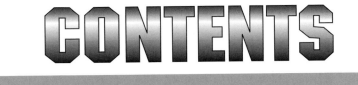

CONTENTS

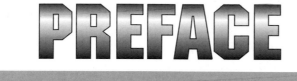

PREFACE

The genesis of *More Muscle* goes back more than 20 years, when I was owner of the original Gold's Gym in Venice, California. The notes I began jotting down on both the practice and scientific basis of weight training had the makings of a book. In fact, I remember the original working title: *Gold's Gym Science of Sport*—a mouthful of pomp and circumstance.

My work at Gold's Gym offered a unique vantage point. The world's most "hard-core" bodybuilders, weight lifters, and professional athletes trained there, hour after grueling hour, to meet their lofty goals. And the few exercise scientists who were, at that time, studying the effects of weight training, followed the champions' every footstep.

Many of the gym members were everyday people, from all walks of life, with more modest training goals. Some were weight training for fitness, some for improved sports performance, some to achieve a more attractive appearance. Yet, however different the training goals for elite and average lifters may have been, all lifters had one thing in common: a desire for physical change.

More Muscle will help you achieve the positive physical changes you seek. If you are a high school or college athlete who wants to improve your strength and power, a well-developed bodybuilder who wants to look even more cut and buffed, or a fitness enthusiast who lifts regularly at home or the gym to get in better muscular shape, this book is for you.

In *More Muscle* you'll find many exceptional features, including the following:

◆ A no-nonsense explanation of why weight training works.

◆ Information-packed sections explaining the capabilities, special stresses, and the care and repair of the weight trainer's body.

◆ Chapters that address your specific training goals. Is it more muscle mass you want, more strength, or more muscular endurance?

◆ Fully illustrated exercises for both free weights and machines.

◆ Sample basic, advanced, and sport-specific lifting programs.

More Muscle is a composite of thc training programs and opinions of those thousands of successful gym members, from Arnold Schwarzenegger, who I saw every day in the gym, to men and women less renowned but equally content with their weight training achievements. *More Muscle* is also a personal statement, based on my 35 years of weight-training experience and a formal education that includes a Phi Beta Kappa key in science.

Part I prepares you for the training programs to come with a foundation of muscle-building knowledge combining practical experience with the latest scientific research. Broad concepts of biology and physics are presented in terms of their significance for the weight trainer.

Part II is devoted to training, both how-to advice and supplementary information that brings the advice to life. Your personal training goals determine which training approach is for you: more muscular strength and power; more muscular endurance; or more muscular mass.

Part III is full of sound strategies for nutrition, weight gain or loss, and injury prevention; strategies that have worked for a generation of champions.

Let me add a final, important point about *you* and *More Muscle*. Whether you want more muscle, more strength, or more endurance, the two most important ingredients in reaching your goals are *motivation* and *expertise*. You've demonstrated motivation by buying this book, which will help you build the training expertise.

ACKNOWLEDGMENTS

Thank you to Ted Miller and Julia Anderson of Human Kinetics for their enthusiasm and editorial assistance.

Thank you to my supportive family: Donna Wong and Kenny, Julie, and Chris Sprague.

A massive thank you to Tom Grace and Gary Jones of Hammer Strength. I greatly appreciate their assistance, along with Sam Doane, creative director in the primary photography work. Photograph credits go to Complete Production Services, Ltd., in association with Photo Design and Kipling Rock Productions in Portland, Oregon; to Speed City Training Facility, where the photographs were taken; and to John Bauguess for supplementary photographs.

Thanks to the outstanding athletic models and their contributions: Wade Blackburn, Chris Green, Dave Hughes, Victoria Johnson, VonRay Johnson, Chanze LaMott, Ember Parks, Paula and Steve Schaffer, Lori Sonneburg, Chris Sprague, Jacque Till, and Marv Wilkerson.

Thank you to the following equipment companies for contributing photographs and state-of-the art information to this book: Hammer Strength, Iron Grip Barbell Company, and Speed City.

A very special thanks to Marv Wilkerson, a long-time weight trainer who knows how to set and accomplish goals, for lending his expertise in the preparation of this manuscript.

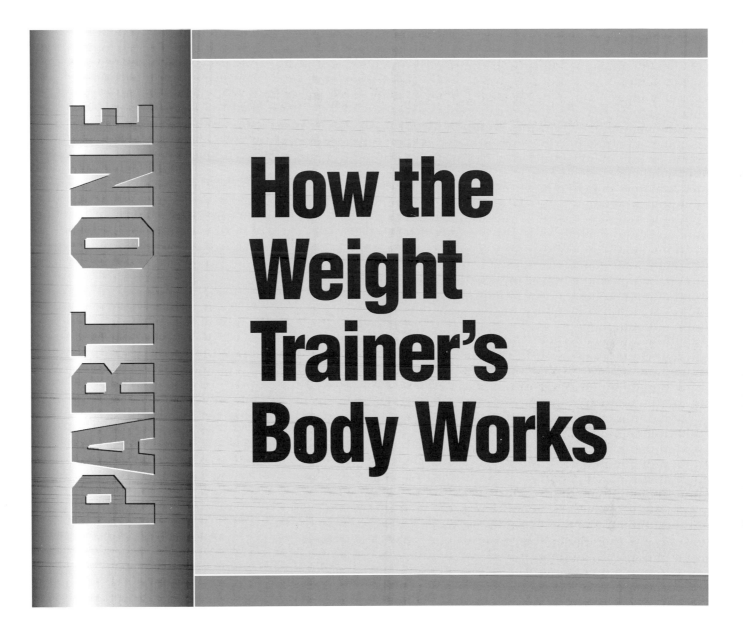

PART ONE

How the Weight Trainer's Body Works

A weight trained body is a complicated machine. It takes in and processes foods for fuel. It gathers, sorts, and acts on information. It sleeps, dreams, breathes, feels pain, thinks up jokes, fends off germs, cools itself, cries, and—of most immediate consequence to the weight trainer—it moves. Moves not just in mundane ways, such as walking the dog, sitting down at the dinner table, or stirring the soup, but also in artistic, athletic movements that engender pleasure to both athlete and spectator.

When we're admiring the grace and skill of a soccer player controlling the ball with her feet, we are oblivious to the myriad systems working inside her. Messages flash along nerves, glands secrete hormones, blood delivers oxygen and nutrients to cells, and muscles move bones. Her body's outward beauty and fluidity conceal a wondrous, flesh-covered bag of guts and gases, muscles and bones.

The old saying that the body is worth only a few pennies if rendered into its chemical components is certainly true. Yet, as an interconnected, biological system, that body can achieve a vast array of physical goals. It's literally priceless when those chemicals have the gift of thought, of movement, of life.

Throughout *More Muscle*, the biological concepts underlying successful weight training are presented hand-in-hand with training advice. But before the first practical tip, let's begin with the foundation of basic muscle science.

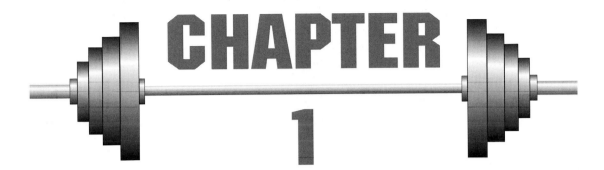

CHAPTER 1

Basic Muscle Science

Sandy Koufax, the great Hall of Fame pitcher, appeared to effortlessly throw a sweeping curveball past befuddled batters. Strike three! No big deal for a big, strong pitcher, right? Wrong.

If we could peel back time and Koufax's skin, we would see hundreds of different muscles contributing to the ultimate success of that curveball. The throw begins as the big muscles of the legs, hips, and torso initiate the forward thrust of body and ball toward the plate. Soon to join the muscular train of motion are the muscles of the shoulder, arm, and hand, creating the twisting forward thrust that gives the curveball its characteristic spin. Too little or too much force from any muscle at any time during the entire pitching motion would send the ball veering out of the strike zone.

Just as with throwing a curveball, the success or failure of all other athletic movements depends on both the capacity and the coordination of individual muscles. Yes, the nervous system, cooling system, and all components of the human machine contribute to athletic competition. But the focus of movement is muscle. "Muscle success" breeds movement success; "muscle failure" breeds movement failure.

Skeletal muscles, the muscles illustrated in figures 1.1 and 1.2, are responsible for athletic movements. They're called skeletal muscles because they're attached to one or more bones of the skeleton. They're the muscles that powered Koufax's curveball, Schwarzenegger's barbells, and Michael Jordan's jump shots. In fact, skeletal muscles are the engines that produce all athletic movements: running, reaching, jumping, bending, and so on. More important, though, is this: The size and performance of your 500 or so skeletal muscles can be improved through weight training. More muscle. More strength. More endurance. That translates to bigger, stronger, faster bodies.

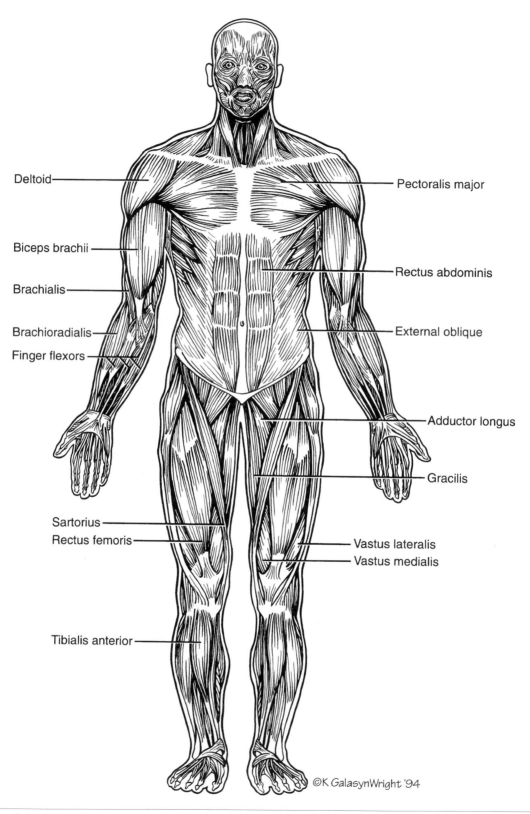

Deltoid

Biceps brachii

Brachialis

Brachioradialis

Finger flexors

Pectoralis major

Rectus abdominis

External oblique

Adductor longus

Gracilis

Sartorius

Rectus femoris

Vastus lateralis

Vastus medialis

Tibialis anterior

©K GalasynWright '94

Fig. 1.1. Front view of adult male human skeletal musculature

© K. Galasyn-Wright, Champaign, IL, 1994.

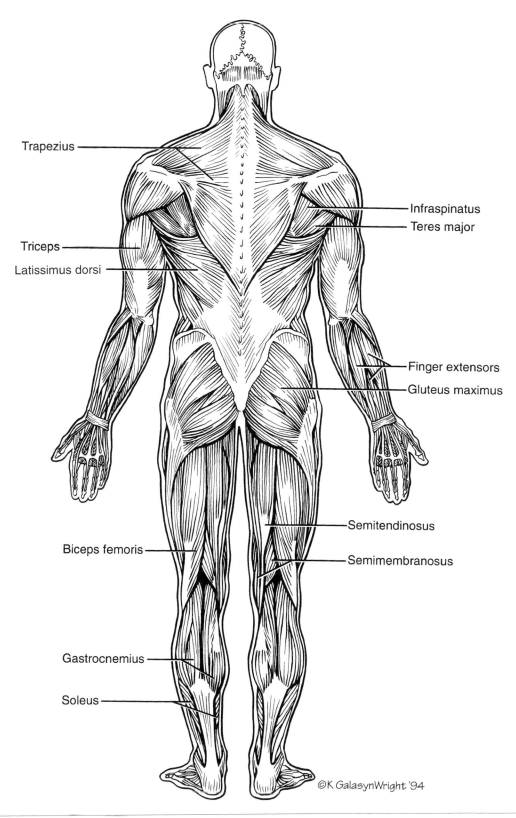

Fig. 1.2. Rear view of adult male human skeletal musculature

© K. Galasyn-Wright, Champaign, IL, 1994.

MUSCLES WORK THROUGH CONTRACTIONS

Muscles work only one way: They contract. *Contract* means "shorten," and that's exactly what a muscle does when it contracts—it shortens in length as opposite ends of the muscle are pulled toward its center.

In turn, the shortening muscle pulls on the attached bones, pulling them together or apart to produce each and every movement. Conversely, movement won't happen without contractions.

Whether describing the movement of one muscle cell or an entire muscle, such as the biceps, the concept of contraction is the same: The one cell or the entire muscle shortens.

In practice, an athletic movement requires many muscle cells contracting in unison. Consider the simple movement of pulling your hand toward your shoulder. Your biceps, one end of which is attached to your upper arm and the other end to your forearm, will do the work. The elbow is merely a hinge. When your brain sends the signal, hundreds of thousands of muscle cells in your biceps simultaneously contract. This mass contraction of muscle cells shortens the biceps, which, in turn, pulls the arm bones together. Voilá, up goes the hand!

Muscles Work in Pairs—One Contracts, One Relaxes

The biceps and triceps of the arm exemplify the natural pairing of muscles. The biceps is the large muscle at the front of the arm that bends the arm at the elbow. Conversely, the triceps is the muscle at the back of the arm responsible for straightening the elbow (see figure 1.3).

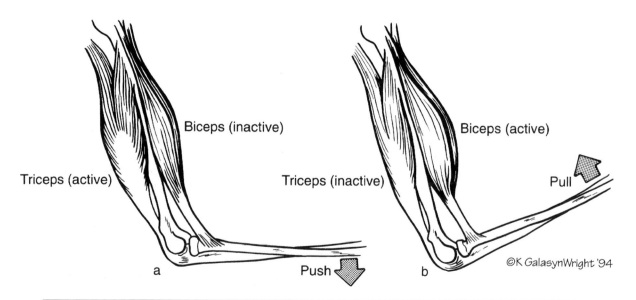

Fig. 1.3. Triceps muscle activity (a) results in an external pushing force, whereas biceps muscle activity (b) results in an external pulling force. During actual body movements, particularly rapid ones, opposing muscle groups are usually both active, although one group predominates.

© K. Galasyn-Wright, Champaign, IL, 1994.

Imagine the predicament of the elbow, caught in the middle of a muscular standoff, if the biceps and triceps simultaneously contract. Movement would cease until the stronger muscle prevails. Fortunately, the body has a built-in mechanism, orchestrated by the nervous system, that prevents any such energy depleting tug-of-war.

When the biceps contracts to bend the elbow, the triceps relaxes, allowing the bend. Conversely, when the triceps contracts to straighten the elbow, the biceps relaxes, allowing it to straighten. Such cooperation is typical of the pairing of skeletal muscles throughout the body. One of a pair contracts; its companion relaxes. For complex, athletic motions like the thrust of a New York Giants lineman or the tennis stroke of a Wimbledon champion, hundreds of synchronized muscular contractions and corresponding relaxations collaborate like dancers in a well rehearsed ballet—all within the split second of an athletic movement.

Sports: A Contractions Numbers Game

Hopscotch to golf, sporting events are distinguished, in part, by the strength, frequency, and duration of the athlete's muscle contractions.

- ◆ Strength events—such as the shot put—demand one to several all-out muscular contractions performed within several seconds.
- ◆ Muscular endurance events—such as a 100-meter dash—demand perhaps 100 medium to strong, quickly paced contractions performed within a time frame of several seconds to several minutes.
- ◆ Cardiovascular events—such as the marathon—demand hundreds to thousands of relatively weak muscular contractions performed over many minutes or hours.

The traditional, generic weight training program—3 sets of 8 repetitions for each exercise—significantly impacts strength development, moderately impacts muscular endurance, and has little, if any, impact on cardiovascular endurance.

Suggestions on modifying the generic weight training program to emphasize either strength or muscular endurance can be found in chapters 6 and 7 of *More Muscle*. What about modifications to enhance cardiovascular endurance? The fact: Weight training, regardless of set and rep combinations, is questionable as a training tool for cardiovascular endurance.

When reading this or any other weight training book, remember that repetitions of an exercise and muscle contractions are one and the same thing. Remembering that fact will make selection of the appropriate combination of sets and reps for your sport an easier task. For now, let's go with the following advice relating to contractions-reps and the strength-endurance conundrum:

- ◆ **Strength:** Weight train with heavy weights and few (1-5) repetitions.
- ◆ **Muscular endurance:** Weight train with high reps (20-100) and moderate weight.

- **Bodybuilding (Mass):** Weight train with moderate repetitions (8-12) and moderate weight.
- **General muscle tone:** Weight train with sets of 10-15 repetitions for a generalized program appealing to the "average" individual interested in moderate muscular fitness.
- **Cardiovascular endurance:** Forget weight training; super-high reps (20 minutes of continuous repetitions) without weights. The object is to increase the heart rate.

THE OPERATING STRENGTH OF MUSCLE

Sandy Koufax not only pitched sweeping curves, he threw blazing fastballs and slow change-ups too, all requiring different force productions by the same muscle groups. Likewise, you and I can do a biceps curl with a feather or a bowling ball: The point is that muscles modulate strength production consistent with the task at hand. Which begs the question: What determines the operating strength of a muscle at any one time?

As noted above, muscles such as the biceps or triceps are composed of millions of muscle cells. The bulk of those cells can—but don't always—contract in unison. The cells that do contract during a given movement exhibit an "all or nothing" phenomenon. That means that the cell either contracts with all possible force or doesn't contract at all.

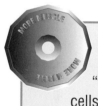

Strength training builds strength two ways. It strengthens individual muscle cells, and it "teaches" more of a muscle's cells, such as the cells of a biceps, to take part in a contraction.

Continuing the example of the biceps, the number of your biceps' cells that contract depends on the work to be done; fewer cells contract when lifting a feather than when lifting a bowling ball. In short, through experience or instantaneous feedback, the strength required is calculated by the brain and nervous system, and then the appropriate number of cells are signaled to contract. Hence, the operating strength of your biceps (or any other muscle) during any movement is determined by:

1. The number of the biceps cells that take part in the movement.
2. The individual strength of each of those participating cells.

Muscle Growth: More Stress, More Muscle

The taller a building, the stronger its foundation must be to endure the stress of the structure. The same holds for muscle—the greater the stress placed on the muscle, the greater the need for larger and stronger muscles to accom-

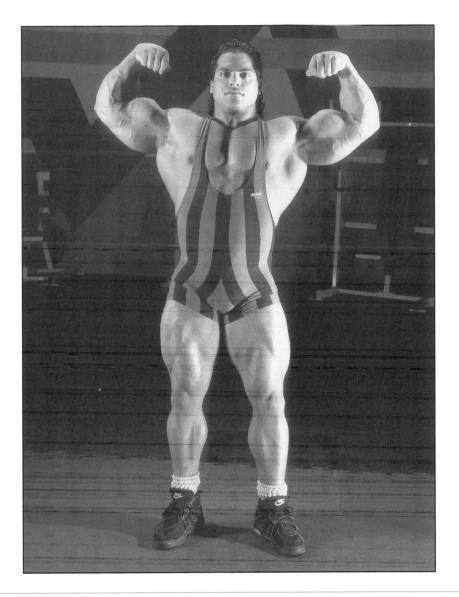

The huge muscular shell is the combined result of millions of microscopic muscle cells continually growing larger from years of adapting to the stress of weight training.

modate that stress. The only (and significant) difference is that architects engineer proactively, building the foundation in anticipation of great stress, but muscles *react*, responding to great stress by building more muscle.

The size of the muscle cell increases as more contractile machinery—long, chemical bands responsible for the shortening action—are packed within. To support that added contractile machinery when the need arises, the muscle stores more energy deposits and enzymes, the complex proteins acting as chemical catalysts in energy production and muscle building.

What about too little stress? The athlete's muscles shrink (atrophy) and weaken, reducing overall cell material, while storing fewer energy deposits and enzymes. The reduction is a natural phaseout of unneeded muscle tissue—the muscle won't foolishly spend the resources necessary to support the excess baggage.

The change in the size and strength of a muscle is merely a natural reaction to stress. Lots of stress leads to a big, strong, buff muscle. Too little stress, and the muscle backslides to its former, weaker self.

Weight training success depends on the muscle's natural reaction to stress. The means of stimulating the stress-response cycle has been codified into the weight training vernacular as *overloading*, our next topic.

OVERLOAD: THE DRIVER OF MUSCLE CHANGES

The conceptual underpinning, if not the exact physiological mechanism, of the relationship between stress, strength, and muscle has been understood for thousands of years. The legendary tale of Milo of Crotona illustrates this point. Milo, a wrestler, lifted his pet baby bull on a daily basis.

Day after day, the bull grew. So, too, did Milo's training stress. The natural reaction to this daily increase in stress was bigger and stronger muscles. Metaphorically, it was self-protection. Milo's muscles armed themselves—with more muscle.

In the gym, barbells have replaced bulls, and the practice of stressing muscles to their capacity has become known as overloading. Overloading is the cornerstone of modern training, whether that training is geared to increase strength, muscular endurance, or cardiovascular endurance. That's because a muscle stressed near capacity reacts through a complex sequence of metabolic processes that better arm the muscle for subsequent onslaughts of stress.

That sequence differs according to the type of overload. For example, overloading the muscle with extremely heavy barbell exercises stimulates metabolic processes that increase the size and contractile strength of muscle cells. A cardiovascular overload stimulates metabolic processes that primarily increase the efficiency of energy utilization within the muscle cell—there is no increase in the size of the cell or the strength of its contractions.

Overloading Builds Bone, Too!

Bulging, rippling cables of developed muscle are readily apparent to the unaided eye, but the bones attached to those muscles develop, too. The most important changes are in bone mass, strength, and density.

The stress of strength training increases bone strength. Weight lifting exercises appear to stimulate bone formation. Like the increases of muscle mass brought about by overload, the increases in bone size and strength are reactive adaptations to stress. Weight training exercises encompass pulling or tugging muscles attached on bones, which keeps the bones strong. The "metabolic processes" manifest as bone-building minerals are added to the existing bone. Minerals (calcium and phosphorus) are added to the bone's exterior surface, increasing the bone's width. Simultaneously, the minerals fill existing open spaces within the bone matrix, the structural fabric of the bone. A thicker, denser bone is a structurally stronger bone.

Weight training also helps prevent bone injuries by improving overall strength and balance, which reduces the risk of falls and consequential bone breaks.

The bone-building calcium and phosphorous, continually

STRONGER BONES AT ANY AGE

Weight training activities benefit bone health and bone strength at any age. Numerous studies demonstrate that this physical activity increases bone strength in children, teens, adult men and women—even those 90 years of age or older.

In one six-month study of fifty people ages 62 to 82 who used a special weight machine that isolates muscles in the lower back, the people increased their spinal bone mineral density by 14%.

circulating within the bloodstream, are readily available and deployable when stress dictates. Like muscle, only those bones adequately stressed increase size and density.

If overload is the foundation of modern training, why don't we just overload our muscles until we drop from absolute exhaustion? As you might suspect, there is a corollary issue to overloading, and that is *overtraining*, an unfortunate syndrome that afflicts both muscle and bone.

Overtraining: Overloading Gone Too Far

Overtraining can be summed up as *too much training stress*, or *too much overloading*. We've already established that an overload is necessary to stimulate a change in the muscle's physiology. Fundamentally, a muscle reacts to heavy barbells, an overload, by growing more muscle. A problem arises when the muscle is again overloaded before the muscle has had adequate time to react to the initial overload. Let's look at the overload-overtraining syndrome.

A strength workout "fatigues" the muscles. Ideally, the muscles "recover" from the fatigue before the next workout. That's why rest days or "light days" (reduced intensity) are a crucial part of an overall workout schedule. With inadequate rest, your muscles haven't recovered from the previous workout when you next enter the gym. In essence, you're overtraining—overloading too frequently—anytime you enter the gym less than 100% ready and able to train.

What's the problem with overtraining? You won't make training gains; your muscles will struggle to hold on to what they have rather than have the excess resources to build something new. In fact, your performance will likely diminish. Your strength and endurance will drop, and the possibility of an injury to a muscle markedly increases.

Bones are also subject to the pitfalls of overtraining. Dr. Ken Singer, a world-famous orthopedic surgeon, explains the frequency of basketball-related foot injuries from overtraining this way: "Every time you are as active as they [college basketball players] are, you injure a few cells. When the rate of injury is faster than the rate of healing, this happens." Whether it be muscle or bone, the accumulation of training stress often concludes with an unnecessary injury. These injuries are analogous to the straw that breaks the camel's back.

As noted above, safeguards to overtraining can be built into a training program by alternating light and heavy workouts. Another strategy is to employ high-stress exercises (i.e., squats and deadlifts) less frequently than low-stress exercises (i.e., sit-ups and curls). Many champion power lifters limit each of the high-stress exercises to one training day per week.

The more motivated weight trainer is often the most likely to overtrain. He or she takes the attitude that if a little training is good, more is better. However, more is not always better; more could be worse. Each weight trainer has a different tolerance and response to training stress. Your goal, then, is to find that individual balance between maximal tolerable overload, engendering maximum gains, and too much overload, which is tantamount to overtraining. That's a tough act to balance: maximal training stress, but not too much training stress.

Finding your optimal overload without overtraining won't happen by chance. One of the best ways of selecting a strategy best for you is listing sets, reps, and results in a training diary. Try different training routines, and evaluate the hard facts from your records. Compare the measured differences and follow a personalized path.

Will you become a modern-day Milo with a 60-inch chest? It probably depends on your motivation. Arnold Schwarzenegger put it best:

> The body isn't used to maybe the ninth, tenth, eleventh, or twelfth rep with a certain weight, so that's what makes the body grow then.
>
> Going through this pain period, experiencing pain in your muscles and aching, and just then go on and go on and then go on. And this last two, three, four repetitions—that's what actually makes the muscle then grow and it then divides one from being a champion and one from not being a champion. If you can make it through the pain period, you make it to be a champion. And if you can't go through, forget it. That's what most people lack, is having the guts, the guts just to go in and just say, I go through and I don't care what happens. And you know, it aches and if I fall down. I have no fear of fainting in a gym because I know it could happen, I threw up many times while I was working out, but it doesn't matter because it's all worth it.

Of course, not many of us find enough value in a 60-inch chest to force our bodies through Arnold's "pain barrier" level of training intensity. Nor will most of us pursue the narrow and arduous task of wrapping our lives around the training regimen necessary to approach a four-minute mile.

The vast majority of us approach weight training more like power walkers than four-minute milers, satisfied with a more moderate level of muscular development—and a more moderate level of training intensity. Life, for most of us, is a balance.

CLOSING SET

This chapter presented the basic structure and functions of the muscles you'll use during each and every weight training repetition. Knowing this basic muscle science will help you better plan, execute, and appreciate your weight training experience.

The potential for a bigger, stronger, or more efficient body is hanging from your bones. All you need to do to realize that potential requires is to overload your muscles beyond current demands. That is the underlying principle of weight training success: Overload those muscles to improve your current level of performance!

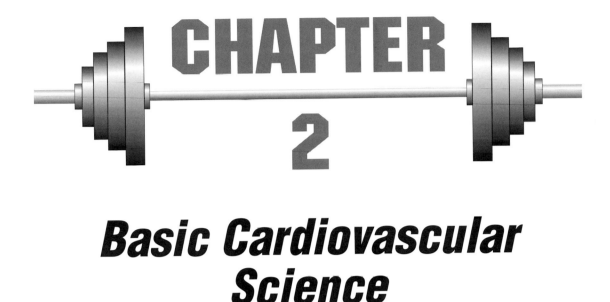

Basic Cardiovascular Science

Weight training improves the strength or endurance capacity of skeletal muscle contractions, but does little to improve cardiovascular performance. Many people do not realize that cardiovascular training is required to improve the strength and endurance capacity of cardiac (heart) muscle contractions. As a matter of fact, cardiovascular training has a great, positive impact on the body's overall energy transport system. Life-supporting oxygen and food more easily reach each of the body's cells—including each skeletal muscle cell. Heart capacity, lung capacity, blood delivery, waste removal, and the body's air-conditioning apparatus are more efficient after a cardiovascular tune-up.

Cardiovascular training has obvious pluses, especially for general health, as we shall see throughout this chapter. Not all weight trainers, though, benefit by including cardiovascular training in an overall workout scheme. This chapter will help you clarify the efficacy of cardiovascular training in meeting your particular needs and goals. We'll begin at the heart of the matter.

THE WEIGHT TRAINER'S UNROMANTIC HEART

The *cardio* in cardiovascular refers to the heart, celebrated by lyricists and storytellers as the body's source of courage, generosity, sympathy, and love; but really the heart is an unromantic, hard-working pump made of muscle.

This workhorse of an organ weighs about half a pound, yet it recirculates your 6 quarts of blood more than 2,000 times a day. Each day of your life, it pumps more than 12,000 quarts of blood—3,000 gallons, or enough to fill a tanker truck—through the more than 60,000 miles of blood vessels in your body. The yearly volume circulated by the heart amounts to enough blood to fill a supertanker.

The heart—already the strongest muscle in the body—can grow bigger and stronger, just as other muscles can. All muscles respond to training in which demands are gradually increased (*progressive resistance training*). There are significant differences between the untrained heart and a trained heart.

An Untrained Heart:

◆ Is the size of a fist.

◆ Pumps with the same force it takes to squeeze a tennis ball.

◆ Pumps 72 times a minute.

◆ Beats (contracts) 100,000 times a day.

The Trained Heart:

◆ Is larger and stronger than the untrained heart.

◆ Beats (contracts) fewer times a minute (30 to 35 beats a minute is not an unusual resting rate).

◆ Beats 50,000 times fewer each day than the untrained heart; it conserves energy.

◆ Supplies oxygen-filled blood to the body with half the effort of the normal heart.

◆ Has enlarged arteries—2 to 3 times larger in diameter than normal—to accommodate the increased blood flow.

A generation ago, many doctors thought a bigger, "athletic" heart was something bad—not much more welcome than a goiter or tumor. Now the medical profession overwhelmingly endorses the health benefits of a stronger, bigger pump, the transportation hub for an ongoing stream of energy, blood, and gases.

Let's focus our attention on a gas, oxygen, and on hemoglobin, a chemical mule-cart. Both are crucial to the operation of each of the weight trainer's cells.

BLOOD AND GASES

Blood takes its color from the solid red corpuscles suspended in the blood's colorless fluid. These red corpuscles are the body's oxygen carriers. More precisely, oxygen attaches to hemoglobin, a chemical compound that is part of the corpuscle. Oxygen first climbs aboard the hemoglobin at the lungs, after crossing one of the many thin-walled blood vessels running through the lung tissue. The oxygen-hemo-globin combo then leaves the lung, traveling along miles of blood vessels until it reaches the cell wall of an oxygen-depleted cell. Here, the oxygen is freed from the hemoglobin and passes through the cell wall into the cell body, where it chemically interacts with carbohydrates to release energy.

Every cell in the body, as it releases energy through this combination of carbohydrates

HOLDING BREATH RAISES BLOOD PRESSURE

Holding your breath during a lift temporarily raises your blood pressure. The pressure from the inflated lungs coupled with the pressure of contracted muscles restricts blood flow in the thoracic section of the body. In fact, researchers have recorded blood pressures beyond 400 mmHg while subjects were executing heavy leg exercises. Do not hold your breath during lifting exercises!

and oxygen, creates a harmful by-product, carbon dioxide, which must be eliminated from the cell. The carbon dioxide exits through the cell membrane into the bloodstream. As in an efficient trucking system, where an outbound shipment of cargo is unloaded and replaced with an inbound shipment, the hemoglobin, after unloading its cargo of oxygen, carries off a load of this carbon dioxide, which easily attaches to the hemoglobin molecule, and delivers it to the lungs.

After reaching the thin-walled vessels of the lungs, the hemoglobin releases the carbon dioxide, which is exhaled into the surrounding atmosphere. The hemoglobin is ready to pick up another load of oxygen, and the cycle repeats.

TRANSPORTING HEAT, THE BY-PRODUCT OF CONTRACTIONS

Carbon dioxide isn't the only cargo passing along the highway of blood. Ever wonder at your odor after you exercise? Ever wonder why a shower is a necessity after a workout? The stink begins because the blood stream transports heat, another harmful by-product of muscle contractions. Muscle contractions produce lots of heat.

Your body functions best within a narrow band of temperature about 98.6 °F. Too much heat can devastate your body. That's why the first probe at the doctor's office is a thermometer: A high temperature is a definite indication of internal trouble.

A performing athlete's body is no different. In fact, if your temperature rises more than 10° above normal during the course of competition or training, protein structures of your brain, muscles, and internal organs begin to slowly cook. What does this have to do with *your* cardiovascular training? Your training attire, your training environment, and the level of training stress affect your body temperature, and moderate variations in your body temperature—less than 2°, can have a major impact on your cardiovascular training performance.

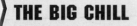

THE BIG CHILL

If the athlete's body temperature drops several degrees below normal, enzyme activity important to all cellular processes slows down. The result is a marked drop in performance along with the temperature. A drop of 10° in body temperature stops even the most courageous heart.

The following are practical tips on controlling your internal temperature when exercising:

1. Dress temperature smart; wear loose clothing or lycra on warm days.
2. Dress humidity smart; wear loose clothing or lycra on humid days.
3. Train smart; reduce training stress on hot, humid days.
4. Drink smart; lots of liquids before and during the workout.

Your body also has some automatic mechanisms to control the buildup of heat produced through a workout of super-high repetitions of muscle contractions. The following sections report on these in depth and explain the preceding advice on dealing with your energy transport system.

Sweating: Purging Heat Energy

Whether it be Shaquille O'Neal romping up and down the basketball court for the Orlando Magic, Nancy Kerrigan spinning around the ice rink, or you pounding along on a treadmill to lose fat before the swimsuit season, the muscular contractions of vigorous exercise produce energy at about the same rate as a 300-watt light bulb. However, most of that 300 watts of energy doesn't add to the strength or endurance of a single athletic movement. Approximately 70 percent of that energy—about 210 watts—is heat, a potentially harmful by-product of the chemical reactions that produced the muscle contractions in the first place.

Let's take a factual (rather than fantastic) voyage inside your body as you move through your cardiovascular workout. The repeated muscle contractions raise your body's interior temperature. In fact, if there were no ongoing means of removing heat, exercising at the rate of 300 watts could raise the temperature of a 150-pound body about 6° per hour. But when operating smoothly, the body is programmed to rid itself of the excess heat energy. Let's explore how that happens.

The heat has no quick, direct exit: Muscles, organs, and other tissues won't allow the heat to easily pass. So the bloodstream comes to the rescue, transporting the heat from the hot innards to the relatively cool surface.

Why is blood such a good transporter of heat? Blood is mostly water, and water is a glutton for heat. Thirty times as much heat can be absorbed by a pound of water as by, say, a pound of copper with the same resultant rise in temperature. Hence, the interior heat is readily absorbed by the passing blood. (*Hot-blooded* should be used to describe cardiovascular exercisers, not people with bad tempers.)

The heat-soaked blood reaches the body's surface, where it fans out into many miles of tiny blood vessels called capillaries. Only a thin layer of skin separates those heat-filled capillaries on one side from waiting beads of sweat on the other.

The heat within the blood can easily cross this thin layer of skin to reach the waiting sweat. The transfer having been made, the cooled blood flows back to the body's interior to pick up another load. What happens to the heat-loaded sweat on your skin? Thanks to another property of water—evaporation—the heated sweat is lifted from the skin. So too is the odor of that sweat.

Your cooling system works night and day, whether exercising or not. You usually don't notice the process; after all, there's no air conditioner humming. Yet when you greatly increase the rate of muscle contractions during a cardiovascular workout, the blood-transport–evaporation cycle can lag behind, even when running on high. The accumulation of smelly sweat is the telltale sign.

Humidity Blocks Heat's Exit

It's no coincidence that Houston and New Orleans were among the first cities with enclosed, air-conditioned stadiums (the Astrodome and the Superdome, respectively), because those cities are among the most humid in America. There are summer days in New Orleans when you can get almost as wet strolling through the French Quarter as you would swimming in Lake Ponchartrain.

Cardiovascular training, lifting weights, or just hoeing weeds is a miserable chore in hot, humid weather. Heat alone isn't the culprit. The body can stand dry heat of 200° F for several hours without a significant loss in efficiency. It's humidity that prevents the exercise-generated heat from leaving the body fast enough. Sweat rolls down your body and dampens your clothing rather than evaporating.

In humid conditions, evaporation is inhibited because the atmosphere is already holding lots of water. For example, 50% humidity means that the air contains 50% of possible water content. Air already heavy with water will evaporate less sweat. At 100% humidity, the surrounding air can't accept any more water (sweat), and your body's cooling system operates with near-zero results.

Cardiovascular endurance activities are affected most by humid conditions. It's not unusual for a distance runner to collapse from the combined effects of heat and humidity. The internal heat generated by the continuous muscular contractions rises and rises until a heat stroke hits. The same thing frequently happens during summer football drills. The football player trains in hot, humid weather with the added heat insulator of heavy clothing, which keeps the heat in, not out.

Weight trainers often compensate for humid weather with

◆ more time between sets;

◆ wearing fewer clothes to allow for better ventilation and evaporation; and

◆ lots of small sips of water.

At the original Gold's Gym in Venice, California, the usual attire to compensate for sultry days was shorts, T-shirt, and shoes (no socks). And the water fountain was one of the most appreciated pieces of equipment.

Whether you're a bodybuilder or marathoner, always compensate for humid conditions in your overall workout plan. Failure to do so can lead to a superheated, inefficient muscular system unable to meet your exercise goals.

The Dangers of Dehydration

Muscle contractions, especially the super-high repetition contractions of cardiovascular training, produce a lot of excess heat, which perspiration helps remove from the body. So sweating is a "cool" part of the body's overall energy transport system. However, removing the dangerous heat can cause another serious problem, dehydration, which comes into play when the body sweats too much.

Anytime the body has less than its maximum water level, it's considered dehydrated. Of course, the degree of dehydration matters. A drop of water lost—unless a tear— isn't noticeable. Losing even a quart of water won't hurt much. Loss of a gallon might cause serious problems for the athlete, though, and during strenuous cardiovascular exercise on a hot day, water loss can be as great as a gallon per hour!

Just a 2% weight loss from dehydration (for a 150-pound athlete, that's 3 pounds, or 1-1/2 quarts) affects the efficiency of the nervous system by raising body temperature above 100° F.

An 8% weight loss produces an internal temperature of 105° F, a higher pulse rate, and symptoms of dizziness and nausea. A 12% weight loss can result in permanent loss of motion by halting the operation of the brain and heart.

To avoid dehydration, drink fluids *before* feeling thirsty, and avoid sugared drinks, which are more slowly absorbed from the stomach.

Dehydration affects all body systems, particularly the energy transport system so crucial to cardiovascular training. The blood thickens from the water loss, placing greater stress on the heart to pump this beet-soup mixture through the arteries. Coinciding with the time of the water-depleted athlete's greatest need, less food and oxygen are carried to the energy-starved cells to replace the energy expended through the exercise. The bottom line is a rapid plunge in cardiovascular efficiency.

That's why you see experienced marathoners snatching a cup of water throughout the race—to stop dehydration before it has a chance to become another competitor. However, there are limits to what the best plans can accomplish.

The runner's body—any body, in fact—can absorb only about a quart of water each hour. This is why high-endurance athletes, such as marathoners, remain thirsty for a long time after exercise; the body is trying to repay the water deficit to the energy transport system.

CARDIOVASCULAR TRAINING: THE BASICS

The mechanism of cardiovascular training is super-high repetitions of muscle contractions. The primary physical adaptations, or physical changes, resulting from cardiovascular training can be generalized as improved energy transport. With those points in mind, the generalities of cardiovascular training can be mapped out.

The basic tenet of all physical training is the systematic increase of stress beyond the customary. If the body is accustomed to curling 10 pounds for 10 repetitions, 11 pounds represents an uncustomary stress; this is progressive resistance training.

In the case of cardiovascular training, the body's energy-transport system is progressively stressed, via the heart, lungs, vessels, enzyme production, and super-high contractions of skeletal muscles. The physical changes resulting from the increased stress are the so-called training effect.

After the body changes in response to the first round of increased stress, the demands are repeatedly increased, over time, through a series of advancing training levels; each successive level is progressively more difficult than the one before. Jogging relies on this principle. Although the jogger's goal is general fitness rather than competitive athletic performance, the training method for accomplishing the goal is the same.

FAT BURNERS

Bodybuilders approach cardiovascular exercises as "fat burners," correctly presuming that the energy expended during cardiovascular training will reduce the body's fat deposits, creating a more streamlined physique. Of course, the strategy works only if the bodybuilder doesn't increase his or her food intake to match the additional energy expended through exercise.

Let's use a hypothetical example, a beginning jogger named Sedentary Sam whose physical activities are pretty much limited to watching TV or walking to the refrigerator to get another piece of cake. Determined to get himself in shape, he spends his first few training sessions walking at a brisk pace (nowhere near the kitchen). After his body adapts to the increased demands, he adds a little jogging. Not much at first—maybe only half a mile out of a combined distance of two miles walking and jogging—but an increase nonetheless. Again the body adapts. Again and again the mileage increases, the consecutive muscular contractions increase, the heart rate stays elevated longer, and the body adapts. Sam becomes a budding marathoner.

The principles of cardiovascular training are always the same, whether the activity is a jog in the park, a rowing machine in front of the television set, a step-aerobics class, or a stairstepper. Those principles are generally agreed to be (a) super-high, consecutive muscle contractions that (b) elevate the heart rate to an age-dependent "target zone" for 20 minutes or more, 3 days or more per week.

FINDING YOUR TARGET ZONE

To calculate your target zone, subtract your age from 220, then take 65% to 85% of that figure. Target heart zone charts are usually displayed on the gym walls, but are also available from the American Heart Association and the President's Council on Physical Fitness. For a quick reference, see table 2.1.

TABLE 2.1　Target Heart Rate Ranges

Age	Predicted Max HR	Target Heart Rate		
		65%	75%	85%
20-29	191-200	124-130	143-150	162-170
30-39	181-190	118-123	136-142	154-161
40-49	171-180	111-117	129-135	145-153
50-59	161-170	105-110	121-128	137-144

Reprinted, by permission, from Golding et al., 1989, *Y's Way to Physical Fitness* (Champaign, IL: Human Kinetics), 156.

Over time, exercise stress is increased by (a) increasing the number of muscle contractions (repetitions, speed, etc.) over the same time, or (b) increasing the duration of exercise while retaining the contraction rate. Does a weight trainer need an improved energy transport system for an effective workout? Probably not. Without the delivery of any new materials or energy, a trained muscle can energize itself for about two minutes, plenty of time for a typical muscle-building set.

There is a mounting body of evidence that cardiovascular training has generally positive health benefits, especially for older people. It's also a way of controlling fat. The latter reason is why bodybuilders monopolize the stair-steppers at the local gym. Cardiovascular training requires a lot of work, self-discipline, and motivation. You could say it takes lots of "cardio."

SUPER STRENGTH AND CARDIOVASCULAR ENDURANCE DON'T MIX

Five-time World Weight Lifting Champion, Vasili Alexyev, often appeared breathless merely from the walk from backstage to the lifting platform. The strongest man alive was near the bottom of the heap in cardiovascular fitness. This illustrates the point that strength and cardiovascular fitness are mutually exclusive qualities. One is measured by a single contraction, the other is measured in thousands of continual contractions, supported by a continuously operating energy transport system.

Optimal strength training and *optimal* cardiovascular training are antithetical pursuits, producing mutually exclusive changes in muscle fiber. The important point is that the heart is best trained with super-high repetitions, and those super-high repetitions impede gains in the strength and muscular endurance of skeletal muscles. Thus, the following advice:

1. *Don't* impede your strength gains through cardiovascular training if your only focus is pure strength or a power event, such as the shot, discus, and weight lifting. Spend your time and energy building strength.

2. *Don't* waste your time with lots of strength training if you're an endurance athlete, such as a marathoner.

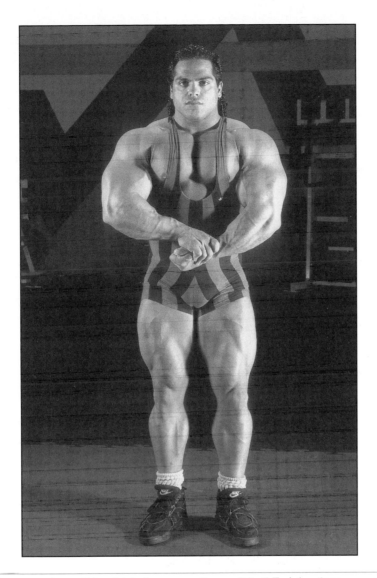

With a quick glance you know this athlete is no marathoner. Why? Training for a marathon—the ultimate cardiovascular activity—doesn't build muscle.

The same concept holds if we toss muscular endurance into the training mix. Simultaneously training for strength, cardiovascular endurance, and muscular endurance—say a cardio workout in the morning, a strength workout in the afternoon, and a muscular endurance workout in the evening—is okay so long as you're aware of the limitations. You can become good at all three, but great at none. Again, some straightforward advice is called for:

1. *Do* spend time mixing cardiovascular endurance with other training protocols if you're involved in a sport with a combination of attributes. Basketball is an example: strength helps the jump; muscular endurance drives the fast break; and cardiovascular endurance sustains the player through 40 minutes of continuous effort.

2. *Do* spend time mixing cardiovascular endurance with strength and muscular endurance training if your goal is general fitness. In fact, if your goal *is* general fitness, read on.

If you're looking for a workout that will *moderately* improve your cardiovascular system *and* muscular strength and endurance, there are ways of combining disparate physical activities to accomplish your goals.

Jogging, swimming, cycling, and skipping rope can all sufficiently raise your heartbeat to achieve your cardiovascular target zone. Combined with a weight training circuit to improve strength and muscular endurance, any one or more of the aforementioned activities provides you with a "cross-training" program.

It is important when combining traditional cardiovascular activities with a weight training circuit to keep the heart rate within the aerobic target zone for 20 to 30 minutes during the workout. Perform each weight training exercise quickly (1 set of 15 reps) and then immediately move on to the next exercise. No slacking, no resting between exercises.

At home, you can combine a circuit of weight training exercises with your stairstepper, stepbench, rower, slide, punching bag, or stationary bicycle. My personal favorite—because I have trouble training alone at home—is the circuit aerobics class at a local health club that combines 20 minutes of step aerobics with a circuit of 10 weight training stations.

BODYBUILDING DOESN'T IMPROVE CARDIOVASCULAR FITNESS

Bodybuilders who don't include cardiovascular training in their overall program have a similar level of cardiovascular fitness as healthy, sedentary individuals.

CLOSING SET

The cardiovascular system is significant not only because it delivers energy to the cells, but also because it removes the harmful by-products of energy production.

Looking at the cosmic picture, we could say that the energy of super-high repetition muscle contractions originates as a stream of sunbeams, speeding across 93,000,000 miles of empty space to Earth. Those energetic sunbeams, converted through the photosynthetic activity of plants and transferred through a food chain, eventually satisfy our human energy needs through meals of chicken, salad, and milk.

However, we needn't dwell on such an immense perspective: How cardiovascular training fits into your overall training goals is more important. I hope this chapter has helped you to determine that.

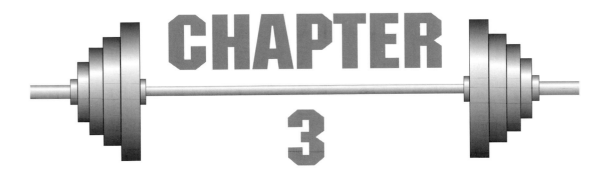

CHAPTER 3

The Mind-Body Connection

Your nervous system, like a vast, biological Internet, flashes electronic messages back and forth, integrating and directing *all* the marvelous physiological activities that actualize your weight training goals.

The neuron, the technical name for the nerve cell, is the "wire" of this communications network. A single neuron operates like a fax with a transmitter on one end and a receiver on the other. Don't let the simplicity of the fax analogy diminish your awe of the human nervous system, though: There are hundreds of billions of these biological faxes sending and receiving messages *each second* of your life. Every sound, sensation, sight, and thought is possible because of our neural Internet. Each muscle contraction—each and every movement—is possible because of our neural Internet.

Given the breadth of the nervous system's involvement in all aspects of your personal biology, it was a challenge selecting the handful of topics most important and informative for your weight training goals. These follow, beginning from the top down with an obviously important topic—the concept of the brain as a living computer.

THE BRAIN: A LIVING COMPUTER

It was the first quarter of the 1995 NFC Championship Game between the Dallas Cowboys and the San Francisco 49ers. Troy Aikman, having called a play-fake in the huddle, threw the ball to the right side of the field.

San Francisco's Eric Davis stepped in front of the ball, intercepting it at the Dallas 44 and returning it for a touchdown. What was going through Davis' head at the point at which he plucked the pass from the air? More than you might think.

Davis' brain, through viewing films and videotapes of Dallas' previous games, had stored in its memory bank all the plays in the Dallas arsenal. Long before Aikman's throw, Davis' brain had stored and interpreted information such as what play calls to expect in similar situations, the wide receivers' usual pass routes, and weather conditions at San Francisco's Candlestick Park. His brain had a database. In other words, Davis programmed his brain with the opposing team's offensive strategy, and his brain calculated probabilities. Aikman's each and every movement was recalculated within Davis' brain as a unique set of probable outcomes.

As the ball left Aikman's hand, nerve impulses moved from Davis' eyes, ears, and limbs to his brain, informing him of such things as the position of the ball, wind velocity, his speed, the position of his hands, and the relative position of opposing players.

As the ball moved toward the intended receiver, continuous sensory input—traveling as nerve impulses—provided the brain with the raw material with which to compute a continuously changing set of probable outcomes. Finally, the brain predicted the position, trajectory, speed, and arrival time of the ball.

The brain's split-second calculations of probable outcomes were matched, micromovement-by-micromovement, to a split-second sequence of orders sent to Davis' muscles. Motor neurons—nerves that signal muscles to contract—controlled the strength, speed, and length of each and every twitch of Davis' body. A successful match of sensory input and motor output sent him gliding off on the intercept path, hands ready to enwrap the ball.

To play the game that well, Davis practiced long hours to gain experience. A brain without experience needs much longer to predict and respond to the flight of the ball. Indeed, for beginners, most responses have to be consciously plotted. With experience, the motions become automatic because the brain has calculated the correct response many times before. The nervous system learns which motor neurons to activate in a familiar situation, a phenomena broadly defined as *motor learning*.

The practical result for Davis is that he performs many actions on the field automatically. Like other professional athletes, Davis has spent the time needed to program his personal biological computer to achieve outstanding, crowd-pleasing performances.

As James Gregg says in his book, *The Sportsman's Eye*, "incoming images are matched with what is on file. The better the file, the more accurate the interpretation will be."

Furthermore, practice teaches the nervous system to connect new combinations of motor neurons—to redesign its network of nerves and muscle cells. If the stimulus for this new network of motor neurons is weight training, the result can be a dramatic increase in strength. A fuller understanding of how this new configuration of nerves and muscle cells increases strength is our next topic.

SMARTER NERVES

Until the 1980s, the collective opinion among exercise physiologists was that strength gains resulted *only* from a combination of bigger muscles and lots of testosterone. That combination described the exclusive domain of adult males. Not coincidentally, before the 1980s, males were also the only group of serious weight trainers.

As large numbers of women and children began weight training, however, that opinion was confounded by evidence. The weight trained women and children gained strength without muscle growth, and testosterone was a nonfactor. Which begged the question: If muscle growth didn't produce the strength gains, what did?

The answer: the nervous system, by rewiring more muscle cells to take part in the practiced weight training movements. As the muscle is subjected to increased training demands, the nervous system "learns" to enlist more muscle cells into service, and as we know, the more muscle cells involved in a movement, the stronger the movement.

As with the growth of individual muscle cells, the nervous system's enlistment of more muscle cells into the strength training exercise is a protective response to training stress. *Neural adaptation* is the name given to the expanded interactions between nerve and muscle cells in response to strength training.

Not only do neural adaptations produce the bulk of strength gains for women and children, they're also responsible for the rapid strength gains of adult males during the first months of a strength training program.

Neural adaptations involve a specialized nerve cell, a *motor neuron*, that connects a nerve to muscle cells. The nerve transmits an electrochemical signal to the connected muscle cells. Upon reaching the muscle cell, the signal stimulates a contraction.

Motor neurons aren't all alike. For example, a neuron serving the eye stimulates as few as ten muscle cells; a neuron serving the calf stimulates as many as 2,000. Whatever the number stimulated, a motor neuron and the muscle cells it signals are known as a *motor unit*. Muscles like the biceps, calves, and triceps are made of many thousands of motor units.

The operating strength of a muscle is determined by the number of muscle cells contributing to a movement. In turn, the number of cells contributing to the movement is a function of the mix of motor units called into play. A heavy load calls many motor units into play; a light load requires few.

How is the appropriate number of motor units determined and called into play? For many activities, experience-coded memory plots an appropriate plan of action. Coded in memory, the nervous system signals the necessary motor units, distinguishing between the requirements for lifting a concrete block or a feather. However, a novel task, such as swinging a bat for the first time, requires immediate, continual feedback between muscle and brain. The quick, ongoing computations select the correct collection of motor units necessary to meet the strength requirements at each stage of the swing. The whole process of calculation and response is instantaneous.

Building strength—for example, learning to lift a heavier barbell—requires the central nervous system (brain and spinal cord) to "rewire." Rewiring, in this sense, means that the central nervous system activates greater numbers of motor units. Over time, through repeated workouts of escalating stress, the rewiring of nerves and muscle is made permanent. The result is greater operating strength, which can be incorporated into an athletic movement to make you a better athlete—without building bigger muscle cells.

TISSUE REMEMBRANCE: RETURNING AFTER A LAYOFF

Watch a child learning to write. Each letter requires a learned coordination between the brain and fingers, input and output. It takes months or years of practice. As adults, we can go months or years without writing a single word, yet the *basic* skills are never lost. The same holds true for the development and retention of athletic techniques. Years were needed for golfer John Daly to perfect his fairway shots and for baseball star Ken Griffey, Jr., to perfect his swing.

Once developed, the skill can be neglected through months or years of inactivity with only a temporary erosion. The reason can be loosely described as *tissue remembrance*, a previously developed biological program that can readily be recalled. Tissue is metaphorically a memory bank; it stores neural wiring schemes that can quickly reactivate physical structures necessary to rapidly reach the previous level of performance. In Daly's case, the precise interactions between feedback loops and motor units necessary to duplicate that fluid golf swing are retrieved from his body's billions of interacting nerve and muscle cells.

As with initial strength increases when beginning a weight training program, previously acquired neural adaptations are the first reacquired in post-layoff training drills. In fact, the nervous system must wait for the physical structures within the muscle cells to catch up with its re-education and rebuilding. The mind is ready but the body isn't—not without weeks of conditioning. That's certainly true of muscle.

Muscle retains the basic structures that generate strength—contracting bands and neural circuitry—throughout the layoff. Many other elements, though, such as enzymes, are in short supply. Returning from the layoff, the stress of resuming hard training reactivates the metabolic processes that resupply the support network of chemicals and fluids necessary to restore the muscle to its previous volume and strength. The process by which muscle volume is restored is conceptually similar to refilling a flat tire: The infusion of renewed air pressure returns the tire to its original shape and function.

To illustrate the above, consider Arnold Schwarzenegger. The famous bodybuilder took many years to sculpt his strong, massive body. Early in his film career, he had to lose approximately 30 lb. of his hard-earned muscle tissue to fit a particular role. His strength dropped, too. What is remarkable is that he regained all that lost strength and body tissue within six weeks of resuming hard training! Although it seems unlikely that a person can lose and regain 30 lb. of muscle in such a short time, the fact that Arnold was on a low carbohydrate diet and measured the same lean-body mass on all occasions indicates the loss-regain cycle represented muscle, not water.

Professional football and baseball players are other excellent examples of a body's ability to quickly regain peak skill and strength levels. After the off-season layoff, professional athletes come to training camp relatively slow, weak, and rusty. Outside their professional uniforms, they could easily be mistaken for weekend athletes. Yet within a few weeks, they play ball as pros are expected to play—quick, strong, and highly skilled.

Professional athletes keep their jobs through tissue memory, reenervating neural circuitry and reinvigorating muscle volume. This sort of tissue memory—storing the basic bits of wiring and superstructure to be later retrieved—shortens your path back to a muscular shape after a layoff.

SYSTEM INTERACTIONS

When Mark Henry, national champion weight lifter, gets ready to lift a heavy barbell, his body goes on alert and crucial changes occur. His heart starts thumping quicker and harder, his blood pressure rises, and his glands increase secretions. You might say his competitive juices are flowing. One of those flowing juices is adrenaline, which interacts with Henry's nervous and muscular systems. Adrenaline, a hormone that is released from Henry's adrenal glands (located above his kidneys), is greatly increased as he approaches the lift. It is not precisely known what triggers the increased secretion of adrenaline in Henry (and the rest of us), but it is generally related to a complex web of psychological effects and nerve reflexes in the cardiovascular system.

Studies do point out that almost at the split-second he lifts that weight, the concentration of adrenaline in Henry's blood increases.

THOSE CRAZY POWER LIFTERS!

Back in the early years of power lifting competitions, before drug rules took effect, some competitors would use a hypodermic syringe to inject themselves with adrenaline before walking onto the platform for an all-out effort.

Sometimes it worked. Sometimes it didn't, because the flush of adrenaline would interfere with the necessary precision of the lift. Invariably, though, the temporary high of the adrenaline boost would be followed by an equally uncharacteristic low as the body rebounded before stabilizing.

When he pulls the weight toward the sky, the adrenaline causes his heart to beat faster and contract more forcefully, thus pumping *more* blood with each contraction! The adrenaline also dilates the coronary arteries, facilitating the increased blood flow.

During what is sometimes an hour-long competition, adrenaline also aids in energy production by speeding up the conversion of glycogen (an energy source stored primarily in the muscles) to glucose (an energy source traveling through the bloodstream) and thereby raising Henry's blood-sugar level. This extra blood sugar is needed by his hard-working muscles. Adrenaline is also responsible for inhibiting intestinal movement during the competition, allowing the athlete's blood to be diverted from the stomach and liver to the working muscles.

As soon as Henry is finished with the competition, his adrenaline surge decreases until reaching its pre-exercise blood level. Blood flow returns to normal, and Henry relaxes, probably with yet another gold medal.

The human body can be viewed as a complex integration of biological systems that can be utilized for what our intellect defines as sport. Muscles, bones, nerves, and hormones all take part. We can separate and examine each system in a book such as this, but in life, they integrate into an inseparable whole.

One last point: Although all our bodies are alike, they are also all somewhat different. That's clear when contemplating the gross differences between 360-lb. power lifter Mark Henry and 90-lb. gymnast Kim Sui. What determines many of those differences—genetics—is the topic of the next chapter.

MOTIVATION: YOU'VE GOTTA WANT IT!

Aside from being born into wealth, motivation correlates highest to success in most walks of life. Highly motivated people reap rewards.

THE CATTLE PROD FOR MOTIVATION!

In my years owning Gold's Gym, I knew several bodybuilding champions who were motivated by a cattle prod, a device that zaps livestock with a painful electric shock. (This is not a joke.)

On days when the confluence of diet and fatigue caused workout intensity to wane, the fear of a zap of the cattle prod from a training partner standing close by resulted in absolute effort during the last reps of a set.

Isn't use of a cattle prod incompatible with the rule that motivation must be self-generated (intrinsic) to produce success? No! Imagine the self-generated motivation necessary to face, set after set, the possibility of a zap of the cattle prod.

Whether intrinsic or extrinsic, this is a training technique I wouldn't recommend!

Like many of life's tangible objects, muscles are there for the taking. Train hard, and they will come. Some people have the requisite motivation to train hard, and some don't. In a nutshell, motivation is why some people will grow more muscle, and some won't. Candidly, neither this nor any other book will help you build bigger, stronger, more efficient muscles unless you're amply motivated to work for them.

Motivation is the need or desire that causes a person to wake up in the morning and attack the day; to work, go to school, or lift heavy weights. On the surface, people are motivated by such things as a

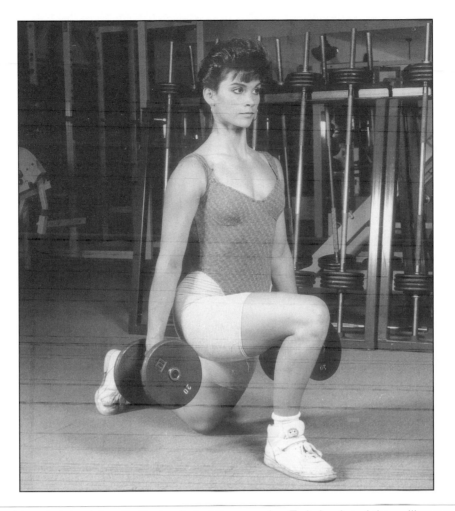

Motivation drives training intensity, the key to building muscles. Train hard, and they will come.

desire for money, a need for fame—or the pursuit of bigger, stronger muscles. Those "surface" motivations often mask underlying psychological underpinnings too complex to analyze and explain in these pages.

Focusing on weight training, less is understood about the dynamics of motivation than the mechanics of growing big muscles. In other words, it's tough to identify the elements that constitute motivation; it's easy to identify the elements of a weight training program. From a trainer's perspective, it's easy to plan a weight training program to build stronger muscles if the athlete comes to the gym with the requisite motivation.

EXERCISE ADDICTION

There is an ongoing dispute over whether addiction is generated by psychology or biochemistry. In other words, is addiction born of neuroticism or reliance on exercise-induced, opiate-like neurotransmitters?

Regardless of cause, the most successful weight trainers—and other athletes too—probably have an addiction to the activity. Especially if we subscribe to the most common definition of addiction as "the condition of being addicted (to a habit); habitual inclination."

Some dated theories claim that sports motivation is a loose manifestation of three underlying psychological factors—aggression, neurosis, and competence. The relative weight of any one factor contributing to the formation of motive depends on the individual athlete and sport in question. A simplistic overview of this psychological hogwash on "drive" finds a boxer or football player heavily motivated by aggression, whereas a golfer might be more motivated to express a need of competence in her golf game. Apparently, there is a lot of overlap in the underlying psychological factors that ultimately coincide to create motivation.

Historically, psychologists dubbed neuroticism as the primary motivation for bodybuilding; the theory being that male bodybuilders (males were the only bodybuilders when the theory originated) were motivated by insecurity or low self-esteem rooted in perceived physical inferiority. In short, bodybuilders were motivated to build an outer shell of rippling muscle to hide a stunted self-concept. But as weight lifting has become a mainstream fitness activity for males and females of all personality types, neuroticism as a collective explanation has lost credence: Yesterday's neuroticism is today's mainstream cultural norm.

It really doesn't matter what generates motivation. What does matter is that *you* are motivated when you enter the weight room. If not—and this is suggested with sincerity—don't expect success.

SUCCESS: EXTRINSIC OR INTRINSIC MOTIVATION?

One of the best motivators for any pursuit is success. Success is positive reinforcement, and positive reinforcement builds habits. That's the case whether the subject matter is mathematics or weight training.

Positive reinforcement from weight training is assured if the first workouts are successful, and neural adaptations virtually guarantee those first workouts will provide positive results. Through neural adaptations, the average person can double his or her strength in a matter of months. That's success. That's positive reinforcement. And that can be habit forming.

Why is motivation so important for weight training success? Because motivated people put more effort into what they're doing. In the gym, greater effort is the same as greater training.

How does greater effort translate to bigger, stronger muscles? Your effort during each set and rep determines whether you're overloading the muscle enough to stimulate physical changes in size and strength. Maximum effort produces maximum rates of change in muscle tissue. Equipment, exercise selection, nutrition, books, genetics—all are *far less* important than putting forth the requisite effort to achieve the stress of a maximum overload.

Maximum intensity is easier said than done. To achieve it demands challenging each repetition, each set, each exercise; in short, an all-out effort. Here are practical tips for operating at maximum intensity:

1. Pick a weight that permits your planned number of repetitions.
2. You'll know that you've chosen too light a weight if you're capable of one additional rep beyond the planned number of repetitions.
3. You'll know you've chosen too heavy a weight when you can't reach the planned number of repetitions. Push the muscle to exhaustion in spite of muscle discomfort. Of course, most people choose an easier path, opting for less than maximum gains.

Motivation, training intensity, and gains are cyclical. Without adequate motivation, there isn't requisite intensity to stimulate change. If you've got motivation, you're going to be one of the quick gainers.

CLOSING SET

This chapter underscores the necessity of interaction between motivation, nerve, and muscle to optimize physical performance.

Initial strength gains are the result of "smarter nerves" rather than more muscle. That's the case whether the weight trainer is male or female, young or old. Only after nerves have exhausted their capacity to rewire does muscle growth become the primary means of strength increase.

The important point to remember is that we can all get stronger, grow more muscle, and improve our physical performance if we have the requisite motivation to follow a consistent training program.

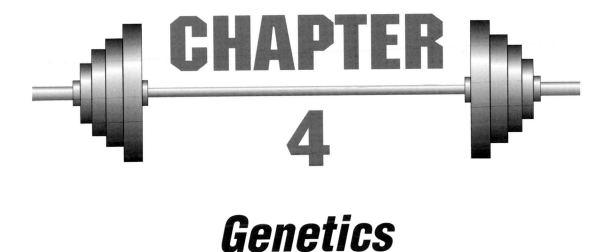

CHAPTER 4

Genetics

Irene Chen, a high school student, won first prize at the 1995 Westinghouse Science Talent Search for a project titled "Expression and Function of Two Novel Genes (PEM and MCAT-2): Implications for Metastasis and Arginine Transport." Her research project isolated two genes linked to lymphoma, a form of cancer.

That a *high school student*, even a very special student like Chen, could formulate and implement such a sophisticated project epitomizes the growth of genetic information. Rarely a day passes that the newspaper or TV doesn't carry the latest breakthrough in genetic research. Genes are a hot topic, an open arena of research! The mere fact that genes have a major impact on our lives—indeed, that they have *any* impact on our lives—is a recent notion, roughly originating with Gregor Mendel's (1822–1884) work on inherited characteristics in pea plants.

Inheritance, passing a combination of traits from both parents to a child, is accomplished through genes. Genes carry characteristics from parent to child, including height, muscle fibers, eye color, finger length, muscle shape, race, and sex. They also carry instructions that guide the baby into childhood, the child into adolescence, the adolescent into young adulthood, and so on until the genes determine that the lifecycle is complete.

Some genetic instructions, such as eye color, have narrowly fixed boundaries and are inflexible throughout life. Other genetic instructions,

CAN SCIENCE OVERRIDE GENETICS?

Sometimes. For example, an inherited gene might program for an underproduction of growth hormone, resulting in a shorter than average child. The child's doctor, overriding the child's inherited genetic program through modern chemistry, may prescribe artificial growth hormone to correct the natural deficiency.

such as those that influence hormone production or intelligence, allow for a range of expression, which is dependent on the person's interaction with the environment. The onset of the menstrual cycle and the wrinkles of old age, as well as the size and strength of a muscle, are other human characteristics that depend on an interaction of genetics and environment. As we will see, the fact that environmental stress interacts with a range of genetic expression is the basis of weight training.

This chapter focuses on aspects of the genetic plan that have the most direct impact on muscle. Let's begin with the beginning: Are the genetic instructions for the number of muscles in both males and females fixed or flexible?

WHO HAS MORE MUSCLES, MR. UNIVERSE OR MISS AMERICA?

Posing under a spotlight and slathered with oil, Mr. Universe seems to have uncountable steel slabs and cables bulging and rippling under his skin. Yet, even counting biceps, triceps, and abdominals, he really has no more muscles than a Miss America contestant who looks as if the next suggestion of a breeze would sweep her away. That's because all males and females are genetically programmed for the same number of muscles, a number that has been developed through hundreds of millions of years of natural selection to meet every demanding movement of which we are capable.

Male or female, we are born with approximately 600 muscles, from the large ones like the quadriceps, biceps, and triceps to the stapedius, one twentieth of an inch long, which controls a tiny bone in the middle ear.

TRAINING PROGRAMS ARE IDENTICAL

Sex-based genetics don't determine the efficacy of training programs. Sex-based genetics determine the relative results of training programs. The only factor affecting program design is personal experience: Beginning, intermediate, and advanced programs in this book are designed for both sexes.

Even the most advanced training methods, nutritional plans, or drugs will not grow one additional muscle beyond nature's genetic package. Of course, you can change the size and strength of those muscles by increasing the size of individual muscle cells, and perhaps add a few new cells, too. For example, bodybuilders often add upwards of 75 lb. of new muscle tissue to an already mature frame, substantially increasing their strength in the process.

We may all have the same number of muscles, but heredity, training, and yes, gender combine to determine how big and powerful they will become. In fact, a more specific discussion of the impact of gender on muscle size and strength is our next topic.

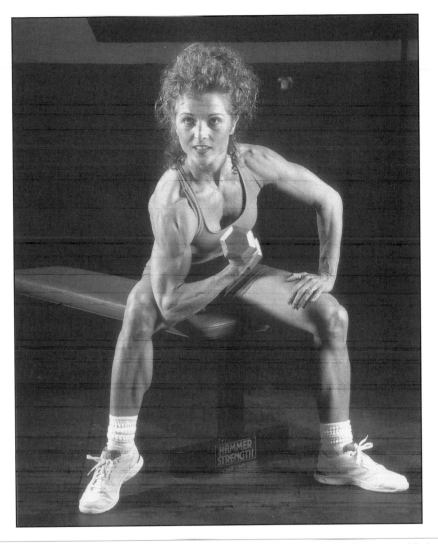

Following identical training programs, an adult female's absolute strength is about two-thirds that of an adult male.

Gender, Structural Differences, and Strength

Compared to adult males, adult females have a tougher time getting stronger. The adult female's absolute strength is about two-thirds that of an adult male's—even if both follow identical training programs. One reason (soon to be discussed) is a paucity of testosterone, but another reason is gender-based skeletal proportions that appear during adolescence.

Until the hormone surge accompanying puberty, boys and girls have a common skeletal design. At puberty, a boys' skeleton grows comparatively taller and wider at the shoulders. Wider shoulders affect strength training results in two ways. First, they create a mechanical advantage for strength, allowing males to exert force through a greater distance; second, the wider shoulders can hold more muscle mass.

Incidentally, strength differences between the sexes is greatest at the shoulders. The difference is much less at the hips, where the female's wider hips offer her a comparative advantage. Enough of an advantage to equal the strength of her male training partner? No, but that's reflective of the testosterone advantage—the focus of our next section.

Boys, Girls, Testosterone, and Muscles

At conception, genes determine whether the child will be a boy or girl. That initial determination is augmented by a cascade of genetic instructions that have a huge impact on the size and strength of muscles. Boys have been programmed for more muscle. You might doubt this fact, though, if you've watched a women's bodybuilding contest on one of the sports channels. Which begs the question: How did *these* women build those huge muscles?

Arnold Schwarzenegger once said about women's muscles: "They grow larger from being trained and fed, just as men's do." That's true to a point: The point being that an average woman could copy Arnold's every set and rep and never grow as big! The primary reason is the difference in male and female body chemistry, specifically the average woman's paucity of testosterone. Undoubtedly, you already know that testosterone is not an Italian dessert. It's a male hormone essential in building larger muscles.

Neither little boys nor little girls produce much testosterone. That's one reason, except for haircuts, clothing, and socially driven activities, children are hard to tell apart. However, hormone production changes with adolescence. Males begin producing more testosterone, females don't.

Testosterone is important for the manufacturing of protein within the muscle cell. In turn, the protein is the raw material that allows the muscle cell to increase in size. Hence, the increased testosterone production at adolescence is integrally related to the male's increased muscle mass at this point in life.

The importance of testosterone to building muscle mass is evidenced by the female athletes who rapidly build muscle mass when ingesting synthetic variations of testosterone. The non–steroid-using female can gain muscle mass through intense training, but the bottom line is that her gains are significantly less than the gains of her male training partner. That brings us back to those anomalous female bodybuilders.

At first glance, female bodybuilders appear to violate the rule regarding testosterone and muscle growth. However, there are two probable explanations for the apparent incongruity: Some female bodybuilders have genetic programs calling for higher than normal testosterone production, and some are ingesting anabolic steroids. Whatever the reason, big muscles on a female are an abnormal adaptation to

ARE FEMALES WEAKER THAN MALES?

Females aren't always weaker than males. Karyn Marshall clean-and-jerked 303 lb. on April 20, 1985; fewer than 1 in 10,000 adult males can clean-and-jerk that weight.

What about the rank and file of female weight trainers? It is not uncommon to find a well trained female 100% stronger than the average, untrained male when both are tested in certain lifts.

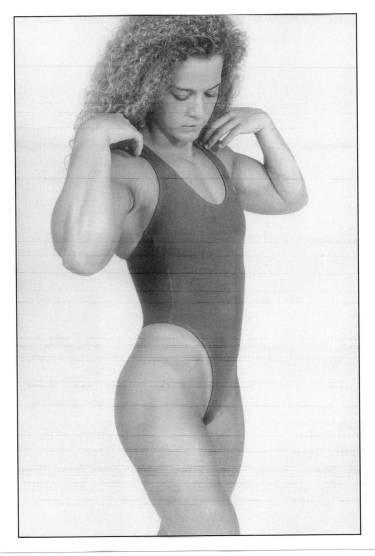

Building muscles is consistent with a womanly body.

weight training. In short, an average female's prospects of building even aver-age-sized male muscles are slim at best.

With that out of the way—that's a lot out of the way, especially if you're a woman hoping to build a Schwarzennegeresque physique—let's turn to a point we've only touched on—same sex differences in hormone production.

All Males Aren't Gender Equals in Testosterone Production

Imagine two training partners having identical training intensity and an iden-tical training program; grunt for grunt, set for set, rep for rep. One partner blossoms into a muscular marvel, the other shows little, if any, visible change. Why? The difference is probably because of different genetic programs for testosterone production.

What you might not know is that testosterone production varies substantially among males. Two "normal" men of the same age can have a tenfold difference in testosterone production. The difference doesn't make much difference in most walks of life, but it does in muscle building. All other things being equal, the testosterone champion will be the bodybuilding champion, and his genes will have made the difference.

Are all other things equal? Another genetic difference is the number of testosterone receptor molecules on the surface of muscle cells. We're all different there, too. Testosterone receptors on the surface of muscle cells are important to muscle growth because the greater the number of receptor molecules, the greater the probability a bit of testosterone will attach to a receptor as it passes that cell. A testosterone molecule attached to a receptor molecule acts as a biological switch, initiating the muscle-building process.

Individual genetic programs for testosterone production and receptor molecules don't necessarily go hand-in-hand. One male might be genetically programmed to produce lots of testosterone but also be programmed for few receptors, or vice-versa. But you can bet that the "quick gainers" have lots of both.

Some athletes attempt to override their genetic program for testosterone production—thus overriding their genetic program for muscle growth—by ingesting steroids. Let's see how that works.

INTERFERING WITH NATURE: STEROIDS

As early as the 1964 Olympics, Polish sprinter Ewa Klobukowska was forced to give up her gold medal because tests showed that her hormones weren't normal. At the Montreal Olympics in 1976, six weight lifters (two of them Americans) were ruled ineligible because they had used steroids, which are synthetic derivatives of testosterone. In 1979, the International Amateur Athletic Federation banned seven women (three Rumanians, two Bulgarians, and two Soviets) for using steroids.

Steroids have been consumed by men in the United States at least since the 1950s, when champion weight lifters wanting to "bulk up" and gain strength started gobbling steroid pills like jellybeans. The news that the genetic program for testosterone production could be circumvented with synthetics quickly spread through the sports world.

How do synthetics pass for natural testosterone? They must "look" and "act" like the real thing under the scrutiny of the muscle cell's testosterone receptor molecules. In other words, the manufactured steroid must have the basic chemical structure and shape

DANGERS OF STEROIDS

In the medical literature, steroid abuse is correlated with numerous physical and psychological problems, from liver cancer and heart disease to infertility and psychotic episodes. Legally, it's a federal crime to prescribe or possess steroids for enhanced athletic performance.

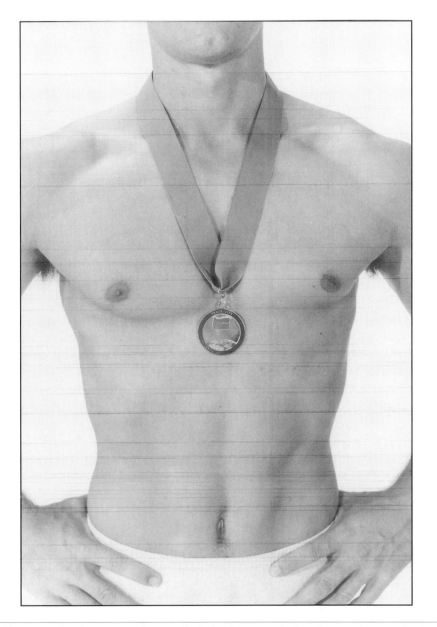

While steroids are a stimulus to muscle growth, federal laws and all major sports organizations prohibit their use to enhance athletic performance.

of natural testosterone. If not a close copy, the muscle cell's testosterone receptors won't interact with the steroid. Steroids are good enough copies to pass the scrutiny of the testosterone receptor molecules.

The testosterone look-alikes, combined with the body's natural testosterone, increase the total concentration of muscle-building hormones circulating through the bloodstream. This greater concentration increases the probability of an interaction with a testosterone receptor molecule—and thus increases the probability of initiating the muscle-building process.

Hormones aren't the only genetic factor affecting the size and strength of muscle. Bone length, skeletal proportions, and the shape of muscles—all factoring into the strength and size of muscles—are genetically determined, too.

GENETICS AND PHYSICAL CHARACTERISTICS

Hormone production isn't the only innate variation that affects weight training success within same-sex groups. Bone density, tendon attachments, muscle fiber type, and muscle shape are a few more inherited physical characteristics having a huge impact on one's weight training potential. Let's explore how and why.

Bones and Tendons: Genetic Advantages, Too

Bodies are genetically programmed for all sorts of shapes and sizes: tall, short; long arms, short arms; broad shoulders, narrow shoulders; big feet, small feet; bird legs, piano legs. The collective human gene pool is an endless diversity of structural combinations, each with a demonstrable impact on weight training results. Let's look at a couple of examples.

We've already seen that gender-related structural differences affect muscle mass and strength differences. Structural differences affect strength and muscle-building potential among same-sex weight trainers, too. The most straightforward example is that a larger skeleton can pack more muscle. A less obvious example is the impact that relative bone length has on strength.

To appreciate the relationship between relative bone length and strength potential, imagine curling a weight placed at mid-forearm rather than in the customary hand position: The mid-forearm position requires much less force to curl the same weight. Likewise, an athlete with a relatively shorter forearm—all other things being equal—has a mechanical advantage in curling a barbell.

Like relative bone lengths, the point of tendon attachment is another genetic variable that has a major effect on strength. Continuing our curl example, a weight trainer with a biceps tendon attached closer to the wrist has a mechanical advantage over a weight trainer with a biceps tendon attachment closer to the elbow.

There's another genetically defined, non–gender-related variation that has an enormous impact on weight training—the innate, highly individualistic ratio of fast to slow twitch muscle fibers we bring to the weight room.

Born With a Twitch, Die With a Twitch

Genetics can carry the curse of a dreaded disease or the gift of gorgeous eyes. As previously noted, genetics also set our potential for strength, muscle endurance, muscle shape, and muscle mass—even muscle "twitch." In short, the genetic lottery greatly influences life's winners and losers.

We're all born with two types of muscle cells (also called muscle fibers), each having distinguishable functional differences. *Fast-twitch* fibers have greater capacity for strength and speed. *Slow-twitch* fibers, which store more energy-producing glycogen, have greater capacity for endurance. What does genetically determined twitch ratio have to do with weight training success?

Athletes with more fast-twitch fibers have greater potential to develop strength and speed.

Research into fiber types fuels the proposition that "lifters and sprinters are born, not made." While everyone can increase strength and speed through proper weight training, world-class lifters and sprinters have a twitch of a genetic headstart.

Although the evidence is generally anecdotal, there appears to be little correlation between fiber type and muscle size; that is, there are very muscular slow guys and very muscular fast guys. Building huge muscles appears possible irrespective of fiber type: 20" biceps come in all fiber combinations. In other words, the potential for muscle mass is apparently determined by factors additional to fiber ratios.

Here's the catch (or twitch): The ratio of fast-twitch to slow-twitch cells is apparently genetically determined. No kind or amount of training will change that genetic ratio. If you're born with a preponderance of fast-twitch fibers, you'll die with a preponderance of fast-twitch fibers.

The good news: Weight training can strengthen what you have, and that added strength translates to better athletic performance. Moreover, weight training can build bigger muscles. Can it change the shape of a muscle, though? The next section provides the answer.

Muscle Shape: Another Genetic Destiny!

Can weight training change the basic shape of a muscle? Absolutely not! Shape, like twitch ratio, is intractably set at birth.

Identical twins—one a weight trainer, the other not—retain identical muscle structure throughout life. If one has a peaked biceps, the other has a peaked biceps. If one has a sweeping triceps, the other has a sweeping triceps, and so on. No amount or type of training will alter that basic structure.

Does that mean that body sculpting—adding a little muscle here and there to balance a physique—is a fraud? No, selectively adding more mass to a muscle of your choice is a primary benefit of weight training. Understand, however, that the added muscle won't change the general structure (i.e., shape) of that muscle. It's analogous to increasing the size of a soda bottle: The shape of the soda bottle remains the same.

Race and Weight Training

Statistical differences can be found when comparing the physical characteristics of different racial groups. Relative length of arms, legs, and trunks, pelvis width, bone density, distribution of and absolute muscle mass, and tendon mass are but a few of the statistical differences.

These attributes can be athletic pluses or minuses. What about bodybuilders? Lee Haney, an African-American, is the only man to win the Mr. Olympia contest more times than Arnold Schwarzenegger. While blacks, on average, have smaller calves, the first black Mr. America, Chris Dickerson, has among the best developed calves in bodybuilding history. The point is that individual genetic programs, *not* race-based averages, ultimately prevail in the athletic world.

Just as there are statistical differences among different racial groups, there are differences within ethnic/regional subpopulations of the same racial group. On a worldwide basis, the best group of distance runners are of West African origin. The best sprinters—including those now living in America—have East African roots.

We've seen that genetics are responsible for countless differences in muscle-building potential. Some are gender-based differences, some are differences within the same gender, and some are statistically race-based. However, all have a wide range of variation—so much so that each weight trainer must be treated truly as an individual, independent of statistical norms.

CLOSING SET

Looking back through the chapter, it's clear that our individual genetic code— even though it is fixed at birth—offers each of us a range of opportunity.

We've found that genetics provide some of us a head start toward muscle-building success. On the other hand, our individual genetic mix rarely prevents any one of us from making startling gains in muscle and strength, if we have the motivation to train hard.

Let's look at the statistics for average males for a rough gauge of the opportunities at *your* fingertips when you commit yourself to a weight training program. The average, untrained adult male is 5'9" tall and 150 lb. The average, competitive, male bodybuilder is 5'9" and 225 lb. The statistical implication: The average male can add 75 pounds of muscle through weight training. That's a lot of added muscle for the average guy!

What about females? Like adult males, weight training will increase the strength and size of a female's muscles. Statistically, they will not reach the same absolute changes in size and strength as males, but they can achieve impressive gains nonetheless. Females commonly double their strength through weight training in spite of a paucity of testosterone.

Are you a genetic wonder that will exceed all previous weight training standards? Probably not. Will your genetic program deprive you of bigger, stronger muscles? Absolutely not. Anyone can improve through weight training— you can bet the house on it.

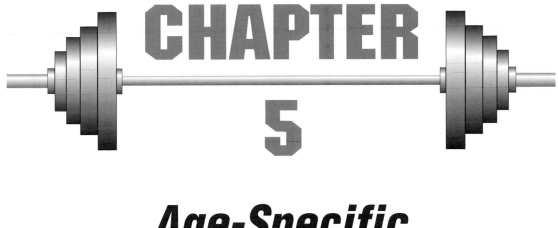

Age-Specific Training Factors

Satchel Paige, the first black pitcher in the American League, played his first major-league game for the Cleveland Indians in 1948. Joining the Indians late in the season, Paige contributed six victories to the team's successful pennant drive. He was 44 years old. Paige appeared in one game for the Kansas City Athletics in 1965, allowing one hit in three innings. At 60, he was the oldest man ever to pitch in the major leagues.

Muscular Methuselahs such as Paige are rare, of course, especially on a pitcher's mound. One reason is that, like maximum muscular strength, the capacity for maximum muscular endurance (referred to as anaerobic endurance) builds to a peak at about age 30 and then declines irreversibly. The 40-year-old athlete typically has 80% of the muscular endurance potential he had at age 30; the 50-year-old has only 60%.

The difference in potential means that the 30-year-old athlete will develop more strength and muscular endurance than the 40-year-old if both follow the same training program. On the other end of the spectrum, Mr. Rookie, age 18, has about the same strength and endurance potential as Mr. Veteran, age 40, but Rookie's potential increases each year as he heads toward 30, while Veteran's potential diminishes with each passing year.

Potential and results don't always follow, though, as Satchel Paige demonstrated. Many older athletes are able to defeat younger rivals because they train harder or because of superior experience or intelligence. Likewise, younger athletes often balance the competitive scales with superior effort.

In this chapter, we'll explore *typical* age-related differences in physiological function. Like Mr. Paige, there are exceptions that defy the typical. We must take the typical with a grain of salt, for no two people age identically.

KIDS AND WEIGHT TRAINING

Kids—or, in technical terms, prepubescents—are packaged in all shapes and sizes, interests, hopes, and dreams, and they grow into adults with the same differing sets of characteristics. Kids may have many differences, but they all follow a similar, genetically prescribed developmental plan. That means that the typical kid is genetically bound to certain age-dependent basic behaviors and physiological functions. For example, the typical child grows 3" taller during his third year of life, after which his growth rate continuously slows, growing perhaps less than an inch during the eleventh year—until the onset of puberty.

WILL WEIGHT TRAINING STUNT A CHILD'S GROWTH?

Absolutely not! Many well monitored studies have overwhelmingly refuted the unfounded myth that weight training stunts growth. My own son, Chris, a 15-year-old 6-footer, has been weight training for 5 years.

Muscle growth mimics the pattern of bone growth, increasing in mass rapidly the first several years then ever more slowly until the onset of puberty. In short, muscle and bone grow in tandem through childhood.

The developmental plan differs little for boys and girls: They remain about the same size throughout childhood. If we set aside cultural influences, athletic performance is similar, too. Ten-year-old boys and girls toss the shot about the same distance, sprint about the same speed, and are equally suited to weight training.

There are five important factors that greatly affect a child's weight training safety and success:

◆ Emotional readiness
◆ Hormones
◆ Stature and motor control
◆ Exercise selection
◆ Sets and reps

Let's explore each of these important factors that might compromise a child's weight training experience.

Emotional Readiness

Emotional readiness is an important training factor. Whether in basketball, gymnastics, academics, weight training, or social interaction, emotional readiness is at once the most important and most difficult variable to assess for children.

The efficacy of a weight training program for a given child takes into account factors such as interest, attention span, ability to follow directions, goal structure, and level of self-control—factors generally associated with the child's cognitive, affective, and value development stages.

Like adults, no two kids are exactly alike. Some will enjoy weight training and some won't. Some aren't ready for weight training today, but might be on another day. The best advice is to *expose* the child to weight training. Adult expectations don't often meld with a child's psyche. You'll quickly learn if it's the right activity at the right time.

POSITIVE REINFORCEMENT

As a rule of thumb, boys and girls 10 and older take to strength training. The rapid strength gains during the first weeks of training provide positive reinforcement toward a sense of competence—and improved self-concept. In short, strength gains reinforce training habits.

Hormones

Hormones affect the *results* of a weight training program. Without substantial testosterone—lacking in both boys and girls—little muscle growth comes during childhood from weight training.

However, research overwhelmingly supports the notion that weight training builds strength and muscular endurance in children. Not just by bits and pieces, but by leaps and bounds: Studies have documented as a much as a 50% increase in strength in both boys and girls after only nine weeks of strength training.

Will the incredible rate of strength increase continue throughout childhood? Probably not. The initial, rapid strength gains result from children learning to use more muscle fibers when attempting a push or pull—the so-called neural adaptations discussed in chapter two. But without hormones to support muscle growth, the learning curve plateaus after several months, and further strength gains are more slowly acquired.

The important point is that, although kids may not be able to grow the showy muscles of weight training, they can certainly become much stronger. This added strength enables young athletes to hit a ball farther, swim faster, or just enjoy the emotional lift of newly acquired competence.

Stature and Motor Control

Stature and motor control come into play primarily in the selection of equipment. There are two interrelated issues regarding equipment. Is the equipment safe and functional in light of a child's smaller frame?

Most exercise machines—both professional models and home units—are designed to fit an average adult's body. That's the case for the full gamut of machines, from single-purpose exercise bikes to multipurpose weight machines. Few can be adjusted to accommodate the size of the very tall or very short among us. Consequently, exercise machines are often inappropriate for the relatively small body of a child. Your best bet is to have a person experienced with the function of the particular machine check its appropriateness for your child.

Free weights, barbells, and dumbbells fit any size body, but even free weights have to be approached with caution. A long bar, or even a dumbbell, can be a bear to balance for a small child—especially when considering a child's relative paucity of *fine-motor control,* the ability to produce finely controlled and coordinated movements. Motor control doesn't peak until the nervous system matures late in the teenage years.

Nothing is innocuous when selecting equipment for a child. A bench might be too wide for immature shoulders. A 5- or 6-foot bar rather than a 7-foot bar may be appropriate. In short, it's a matter of fit.

Exercise Selection

Exercise selection is more a matter of experience than of age. Until the child is experienced with equipment, technique, and gym protocol, all exercise selection is suspect. Particularly suspect is the inclusion of overhead lifts into the child's training program.

Overhead lifts provide the greatest potential for serious trauma: The weights have farther to fall before hitting a head or toe, and the exercise requires more balance and technical expertise than most other weight training exercises. The skills required for overhead lifts are gradually acquired through the experience of having mastered other, less problematic, exercises. That's the case whether the lifter is an adult or child.

A rule of thumb: The child's program should not include overhead lifts until that child has had several years of lifting experience. Refer to an earlier book I coauthored with Chris Sprague, *Weight and Strength Training for Kids and Teenagers* (1991), for more in-depth training information and a review of science research on this topic.

Sets and Reps

Sets and reps must be modified for the child. The numerous sets that an adult bodybuilder performs would stress the average child both emotionally and physically to the point of wanting to avoid all contact with weight training. A father or mother pushing a child to that point is, quite frankly, abusing the child.

The reasonable approach is to start small and allow the child to increase the program at his or her comfort. A small start might include the following:

◆ 2 sets of 12 to 15 reps per exercise.

◆ 6 to 8 exercises per workout.

◆ 2 or 3 workouts per week.

As much as possible, be the brake rather than the accelerator. Supplement the child's enthusiasm with adult judgment, support, and expertise.

In conclusion, is weight training safe for a child? Yes, *if* the child performs a program designed for a child, and *if* the child is supervised by an experienced adult. That might seem like two big "ifs," but it's not meant to be a turn-off. There is no evidence whatsoever that children are at an increased risk of injury from a properly executed weight training program. In fact, statistics reflect that children are injured less frequently during weight training than during other typical childhood fitness activities such as gymnastics, running, wrestling, basketball, and soccer.

The keys to physical safety are *adult supervision* and a *specially designed program* encompassing the experiential and physical factors of childhood which were addressed above.

ADOLESCENCE: THE GROWTH SPURT

Adolescence is a maturational benchmark, separating child from adult. For most kids, that benchmark is reached between ages 12 and 15 for boys and 10 to 13 for girls. With adolescence comes the *growth spurt*, a sudden surge in height taking place after height increases all but stopped during childhood.

There are rapid internal changes to body chemistry, too. Glands produce a surge of gender-specific hormones, producing the secondary characteristics— voice, muscularity, facial hair, muscle mass—differentiating the physical characteristics defining "masculine" and "feminine."

Typically, interest in weight training—especially among boys— skyrockets at adolescence. This skyrocketing interest in a heretofore untested activity, coupled with a rapidly changing body, impacts both the design and results of a weight training program. A discussion of the most important issues surrounding that impact follow.

Early Adolescence: Emphasize Safety

Most often, the child is in middle school when the adolescent switch turns on. Growth quickens, and males usually begin to pay more attention to their muscles. It's also a time when males' "raging hormones," a phrase familiar to middle school teachers, heighten the possibility of less-than-rational conduct and body odor.

Not coincidentally, middle school is typically the first time that young boys weight train. Hence, the image of the typical middle schooler is one with great exuberance, little judgment, and no weight training experience. This typical combination of factors increases the potential for injury. Safety requires that the middle schooler's exuberance be supplemented with an adult's judgment and experience. In short, experienced adult supervision is needed to ensure a safe training environment.

This is not to say that the middle schooler will maim himself if left unattended with a set of weights. Overwhelmingly, accidents fall into the category of smashed fingers and toes—injuries sustained during other adolescent physical activity. Nevertheless, in all settings, from swimming to weight training, supervision reduces the possibility of these minor injuries.

The best advice: When you present your child with a set of barbells or a gym membership, plan on spending time to teach and instill habits conducive to safe use.

Protecting the Growth Spurt

At its peak, the *growth spurt* translates to four inches of height a year for the typical boy, and three inches for the typical girl. Three issues derivative of this rapid growth must be addressed:

◆ Avoid maximal weights.
◆ Focus on abdominals and lower back.
◆ Accommodate for decreased flexibility.

Let's take them one at a time.

Avoid Maximal Weights

The American Academy of Pediatrics recommends that maximal weights not be lifted until the weight trainer has reached his or her 16th birthday. That's the typical age at which 99% of adult height has been reached, a time when the growth spurt is past.

Before adult stature is reached—particularly during the growth spurt—the skeleton's growth centers (growth plates) are thought to be particularly subject to injuries which could blunt skeletal growth. Dropping a dumbbell or barbell on a growth plate is the most obvious means of growth plate injury. The same type of injury could as easily be sustained from a fall off the playground's monkey bars or a tumble from a bicycle.

Another possibility of a skeletal injury results from repeated microtraumas of lifting heavy weights. No single, distinguishable, dropped weight or bump that injures; just lots of high stress pushes and pulls that, in total, adversely impact skeletal growth. In a sense, it's analogous to that final straw that breaks the camel's back.

The important point to remember is that the safe use of maximal weights depends on the individual weight trainer having reached skeletal maturity. Until that time, avoid trying to lift the maximum you can manage; rather, stick with a weight that you can lift for 8 to 12 repetitions.

Focus on the Abdominals and Lower Back

Regardless of age, most trainers suggest a year of abdominal and lower back strengthening exercises before starting squats and overhead lifts. That's particularly good advice for adolescents.

Adolescence is a perfect time to build a torso strength-base, in anticipation of squats and overhead lifts to come later in a weight training program. A strong lower back and abdomen is a boon to sports: It acts as a conduit for the power generated by the large muscles of the hips and legs to reach the shoulders and arms.

In short, strengthening the lower torso makes a better athlete while protecting from unnecessary injuries now and in the future.

Accommodate for Decreased Flexibility

In childhood, muscle and bone grow in tandem. A little bone growth is accompanied by a little muscle growth. Flexibility isn't compromised.

However, with the onset of the adolescent growth spurt, the three to four inches of bone growth per year stretches the muscles' capacity to keep up. In other words, the bone length increases faster than muscle length.

The result of the inequity in growth rates is a loss of flexibility, especially in the hamstrings (back of thigh) and spinal erectors (along the spinal column from hip to neck). Taken together, the tight hamstrings and spinal erectors exaggerate the forward curvature of the lower spine, increasing the risk of injury to the lower back—particularly when coupled with squats and overhead lifts.

The bottom line: Include flexibility exercises in the adolescent's training program, avoid overhead lifts and squats, and strengthen the abdominals and lower back as a safety net.

Sometimes adolescents, not unlike the rest of us, opt for instant gratification at the expense of long-term rewards. If that instant gratification is big muscles through steroids, there is a potential for long-term, deleterious effects on body and mind.

Steroids and the Growth Spurt

Steroids are sometimes the target of media sensation. Overly dramatic anecdotes chronicle the physical disasters precipitated by steroids, even when no credible evidence substantiates the claims in question. It's not hard to understand why some weight trainers pass off all negative attention given steroids as just another phony gambit to increase ratings share.

Nevertheless, the potential deleterious effects of steroids on adolescent skeletal growth is not just more media hype. In fact, the strongest medical argument against adolescent steroid use concerns the potential impact on normal growth and development.

STEROIDS AFFECT THE MIND, TOO

Steroids have been reported to cause psychotic episodes in otherwise healthy adolescents. These episodes are examples of the "roid rage" that has captured the media's attention. Whatever the term, the chemical imbalances produced by the ingested steroids appear to contribute to a group of aggressive, negative behaviors.

Simplistically, steroids are manufactured copies of testosterone. Beginning in adolescence large quantities of testosterone are naturally produced by the male's endocrine system. There is no doubt that testosterone has a positive impact on the adolescent's growth and development. How does adding a little more testosterone (via steroids) hurt?

The adolescent's endocrine system is a finely tuned hormone production system, releasing testosterone in harmony with many other hormones, operating through a series of checks and balances. A *little more* artificial testosterone imbalances the system.

In fact, the testosterone substitutes (steroids), combined with natural production, amount to a flood of testosterone. This flood of testosterone saturates the receptors on the muscle cells, stimulating protein synthesis and the desired muscle growth. However, bones also have testosterone receptors. Unfortunately, the testosterone receptors in the bone's growth plates are saturated by this unnatural flood. Saturation is a signal for the growth plates to fuse into bone. Once fused, skeletal growth ceases.

How much potential height is lost from steroid use is unknown. That probably depends on the quantity and length of steroid use. One point is certain: There is *no* positive benefit on skeletal growth.

Past the Growth Spurt, No More Modifications

Once past the growth spurt, the young man or woman can forget age related program modifications. The only other modifications relate to individual experience and abilities.

One important point for athletes of any age: Carefully consider the relevance of a program for your individual goals. Don't follow a famous bodybuilder's program if your goal is to increase your strength for the shot put. Follow a shot putter's training program. In other words, don't be a generalist; be specific in your goals and follow the most direct path to those goals.

The basic training information in *More Muscle* is aimed at adults of traditional peak performance age, 18 to 30. We've considered special circumstances for kids and adolescents.

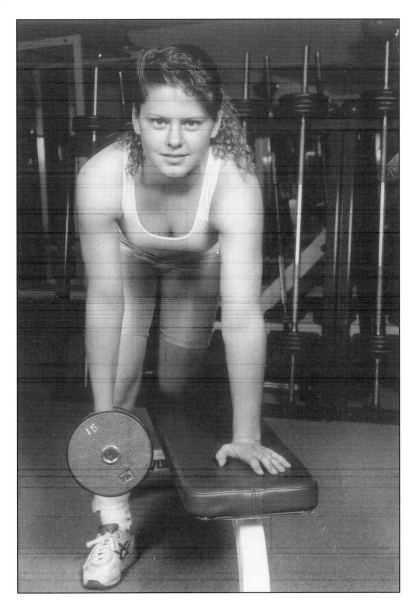

After adolescence, train like an adult: Individual experience, ability, and specific goals are the only reasons to modify training programs.

PROFILE: MARV WILKERSON

Marv Wilkerson is a 61-year-old education administrator who has been weight training for 45 years. Regardless of your age, you and he doubtless have much in common.

Marv started weight training when, as a 125 pound, 16-year-old high school junior, he wanted to be bigger and stronger. With the proceeds of a World War II bond given to him by his grandmother, he purchased his first set of Joe Weider barbells.

The next step was putting together a gym. Weight training was discouraged at school, and there was no commercial gym in Marv's home town (Santa Rosa, California). In fact, few towns could boast of having a weight training gym in the 1950s. Hence, Marv and a few buddies converted an old garage behind his house into a makeshift gym. Squat racks and benches were made of wood; blankets were tossed atop the benches to protect from splinters.

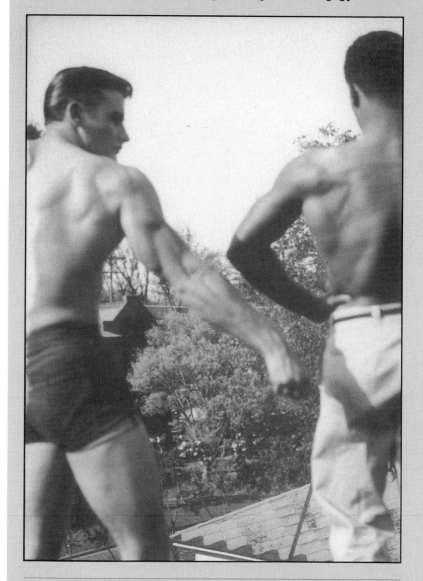

Even if coaches of the time frowned on weight training, the kids had other thoughts. The garage gym quickly became a mecca for athletes, particularly shot putters and discus throwers who soon became local champions. What about Marv?

Marv gained 50 pounds during his first year of weight training, growing from 125 to 175 pounds body weight. Remarkably, he gained only one inch on his waist, from 27 to 28 inches. In short, he gained lots of muscle and strength: He had achieved the goals that had motivated his initial interest in weight training.

After high school, Marv went to the University of California at Berkeley, receiving an MA on a scholarship. He would later earn a doctorate.

Marv Wilkerson (left), circa 1950, as a muscular teenager after having gained 50 pounds of muscle in one year of weight training.

Along the way, with the obligations of family (three daughters) and school, weight training had to take a back seat. The barbells gathered dust in a series of garages as he traveled from campus to campus.

With college complete, and secure in an occupation, Marv was again bitten by the "iron bug." This infection, though, was much different than that of his teenage years. He built a complete home gym of the latest machines and free weights, and health replaced "bigness" as his primary goal (although he admits to going through some "ego periods" where he has used heavier weights).

At 61 years old, what is Marv's approach to working out? "A workout is an integral part of my life. I work out 4 to 6 days a week. I always do abs first because I don't like to do them."

"I see that what the magazines advocate now—the basics—are what I've been doing all along. I have no illusion about having younger joints, so I don't do direct isolation, single-joint exercises. My joints don't have the lubrication like they used to, so I do multiple joint exercises."

Most important is the mind-set with which Marv enters the workout: "After I close the gym door and turn on the radio, nothing interferes with my workout. Jesus Christ or Mary Magdalene might call, but I won't answer. Nothing interferes with my workout."

Marv is a great guy who has accomplished a lot in his professional life. As an avocation, he has learned everything there is to know about weight training. Considering his 45 years of weight training experience, you would be well served to seriously consider his workout routine.

PUSH AND PULL PROGRAM

Muscle group	Exercises	Sets	Reps	% of weight used Heavy	Light	Days/week
Pectorals	Bench Press	4-5	6-8 (light) 3-6 (heavy)	90	80	M/Th/Sa
Pectorals	Close Grip Bench Press	3	6-8 (light) 5 (heavy)	90	80	M/Th/Sa
Deltoids, triceps	Push Press	3	6-8 (light) 5 (heavy)	90	80	M/Th/Sa
Deltoids	Upright Rows	3	6-8 (light) 5 (heavy)	90	80	M/Th/Sa
Latissimus dorsi	Bent-Over Barbell Rows	3	6-8 (light) 5 (heavy)	90	80	M/Th/Sa
Biceps	Barbell Curl	3	8-10 (light) 6-8 (heavy)	90	80	M/Th/Sa

LEGS PROGRAM

| Muscle group | Exercises | Sets | Reps | % of weight used | | Days/week |
				Heavy	Light	
Quadriceps, erector spinae	Deadlift	2	8		80	W
Quadriceps	Squats	4-5	6-8 (light) 5 (heavy)	90	80	W
Quadriceps	Leg Press	4-5	10 (light) 8 (heavy)	90	80	W
Hamstrings	Leg Curl	2	8-10		80	W
Calves	Calf Raise	3	15	90		W

ABDOMINALS PROGRAM

Muscle group	Exercises	Sets	Reps	Days/week
Abdominals	Hanging Leg Raises	3	25	M/W/Th/Sa
Abdominals	Crunches	3	25	M/W/Th/Sa

WEEKLY SCHEDULE

Monday	Tuesday	Wednesday	Thursday	Friday	Saturday	Sunday
Push and Pull Abdominals	REST	Legs Abdominals	Push and Pull Abdominals	REST	Push and Pull Abdominals	REST

Note. *The abdominal workout is done prior to the other weight training program each day. These are all basic exercises (no isolation ones). The Push and Pull Program takes about 45 minutes, and the Legs Program takes about 25 minutes.*

GETTING OLDER (THAN 30)

It's no secret—in fact it's impossible to hide—that human performance peaks at about age 30. Past that point, all physiological functions take a slow, downhill slide. It's "over the hill," Bub. What a sentence-stopping thought for a 50-year-old writer, namely me!

On the other hand, I can take relative solace in the statistical fact that I'm still stronger and carry more muscle than 99% of 33-year-olds. Not as massive and strong as I was at 30, but more massive and stronger than I would have been had I never trained.

That's what aging is all about—it's a personal, nondiscriminatory slide from peak physiological function. Albeit a relative slide: Those starting higher on the slide will remain, relative to baseline performance, higher on the slide.

Can the decrease in performance be partially abated through training? Certainly. Lou Ferrigno, now in his mid-40s, carries 300 pounds of muscle at 3% body fat. That's 35 pounds more muscle and less body fat than he carried in his 20s, when he won the Mr. Universe contest. That's getting ahead of the story, though. Let's begin with some rough statistics, like how slick the typical slide is.

Rate of Decline

During the four decades from ages 30 to 70, *all* physiological functions decline at roughly the rate of 0.75 to 1.0% per year. Over the 40-year period, that translates to a decline of roughly 30 to 40% from peak performance. "It feels like more," you might say.

On the other hand, you might ask, "Is a 30 to 40% decline in physiological function inevitable?" Probably not. Much statistical evidence suggests that the degree of a person's function loss is somewhat dependent on his overall health practices, including physical activity.

A correlation between a healthy lifestyle and a smoother, more efficiently operating body makes common sense, too. For example, a weight trainer who continues to overload his muscles through his 30s, 40s, 50s, 60s, and 70s will retain more strength than a sedentary person who avoids muscular stress at every opportunity.

The correlation between lifelong overload and function retention holds for all physical functions: flexibility, cardiorespiratory function, strength, and muscular endurance. Even mental processes appear

SLOW DOWN NATURAL MUSCLE LOSS PROCESS BY STRENGTH TRAINING

For each decade of life, the average adult loses approximately 5 to 7 lb. of muscle. To prevent this, regular strength training can add about 3 lb. of muscle mass within two months. Research studies of men and women from ages 60 to 90 showed that 8 to 12 weeks of consistent weight training increased not only their muscular strength but also increased their muscle size by 10%.

to retain vim and vigor when consistently challenged. In other words, use it and you'll lose less of it.

A long-time friend, Kent Kuehn, didn't begin weight training until he was nearly 30 years old. At 40, he won the Over-40 Mr. America and Mr. Universe contests. Kent didn't just hold on to what he had at 30, which wasn't a contest-winning physique. At 40, he was much bigger and stronger than at any previous time in his life.

Is Kent's story merely an example of a statistical aberration? No. Muscle mass and strength continue to increase well past 30—*if* subjected to the stress of overload training. In other words, 30-year-olds need not be the baseline of maximum muscular performance.

Why? Apparently, the muscles' rate of adaptation to stress—growing bigger and stronger—is greater than rate of age related physical decline. Not until well beyond 30 do the cumulative effects of age related decline outpace the rate of stress related adaptation. All this is another way of saying that you can be bigger and stronger at 40 than at 30, if you have the motivation to train hard and stick with the training. Of course, there can be obstacles along the way that interfere with the most motivated weight trainers. On a sour note, let's talk about a common age related obstacle to most athletic participation—degenerative joint diseases.

Oh, Those Aching Joints

Longtime, hardcore bodybuilders suffer their share of degenerative joint disease, but they're not alone in the affliction. Top-flight basketball and football players suffer through the same aching joints as they hobble toward their rockers.

On the other hand, athletes aren't the only subpopulations of old people with joint problems. Upwards of 80% of adults between 55 and 64 show signs of osteoarthritis in at least one joint. The statistics beg two questions. Is there any way to train to avoid joint problems later in life? Is there any way of lessening the agony of existing joint problems?

The potential for joint problems increases with trauma and ballistic movements involving the joint. That's why the incidence of arthritis is rampant among retired football and basketball stars whose joints, over the years, repeatedly endured every conceivable bump, grind, and bounce. Analogously, weight

SENIORS IN THE GYM

As a result of recently published scientific studies linking weight training and improved strength, balance, and coordination, health clubs and hospitals have found a new market niche: senior citizens. In many gyms and hospital therapy rooms, personal trainers and physical therapy staff have implemented new fitness programs specifically designed for mature people over 55 years of age. They guide seniors through a variety of weight training exercises to ensure bone building throughout the body. Because the benefits of weight-bearing exercise are site-specific, areas prone to injury, such as ankles and wrist, are emphasized in a senior's workout program.

trainers who train too often (without adequate recuperation), or with ballistic rather than controlled movements, are subject to much the same risk. Hence, the advice to reduce risk is:

1. Control the exercise movement: Don't unnecessarily bounce or accelerate through a movement.
2. Don't overflex or hyperextend an exercise movement.
3. Above all, don't overtrain (see "Overtraining," pg. 11).

What about lessening age related symptoms of arthritis? There's good news. Exercising the joints through a properly designed weight training program apparently impedes the advance of the ravishes of arthritis while increasing joint flexibility. Of course, the same proscriptions regarding overtraining and ballistic, overflexed, and hyperextended movements that apply to the younger lifter apply to the older lifter as well.

The evidence indicates that you're better off trading in the cane and rocker for a barbell and squat rack.

Does Flexibility Drop With Advancing Age?

There is no conclusive evidence that aging, per se, causes a decrease in flexibility. Lack of use causes a loss of flexibility.

As a person gets older, he or she often abbreviates common, everyday movements. It's human nature to take the path of least resistance, and a less resistive path is readily available in a modern environment of automobiles, remote controls, and elevators. All these modern devices *require less muscle power* than their historical predecessors.

How does an environment requiring less muscle power relate to a loss of flexibility? Let's look to the legs for an example.

The legs are the first to lose both strength and flexibility because full leg movements use lots of muscle, which requires lots of effort. We find ourselves bending over at the waist to fetch the morning newspaper rather than more strenuously bending down at the knees. The result is a knee joint that is rarely put through a full range of motion during the course of a typical day and thus loses both strength and flexibility over time.

The good news is that weight training the joint through a full range of motion will increase strength *and* flexibility. That's another reason to incorporate complete movements into your weight training workout. Yes, full movements—especially squats and leg presses—are tougher than their abbreviated

BEGINNING LIFTERS: USE FULL MOVEMENTS!

A detrimental habit of many beginners—young or old—is partial movements, particularly squats. That's because partial squats are easier than full squats. If you want to insure long-term flexibility while getting the most from your exercise time, get in the habit of full movement exercises.

versions, but the full movement is the only way of ensuring maximum flexibility. In other words, whatever your paper-fetching habits, follow the path of greatest resistance in the gym even if you dread those full movements. It's the right routine for your future years of health.

That's enough said about special training factors relating to the past-30 set. As you saw, there really isn't much difference in training protocol when comparing the 50-year-old to the 30-year-old. So let's conclude by reiterating the focal points gleaned from the previous section for the past-30 set:

◆ Beginners of all ages should proceed with caution.

◆ Accept natural limitations. Don't compete with the past.

◆ As age increases, coordination decreases. Machines are generally safer than free weights when coordination is a problem.

◆ Avoiding ballistic movements will help avoid joint pain now and later.

◆ Avoid partial movement exercises—exercise the muscle through a full range of motion.

◆ Don't overtrain.

◆ The most important point to remember is that all adults respond to weight training more or less the same. Perhaps advancing age statistically limits absolute strength and mass, but an individual's strength and mass can increase well past 30 if he or she continues to weight train.

CLOSING SET

Young, old, or in between, weight training has positive advantages as a fitness activity. All ages can experience a stronger, more flexible body through weight training.

Individual differences in programs depend on experience and baseline ability. Exercise selection and resistance levels should reflect the individual's familiarity with the weight room, maturational stage, and individual physical capacity.

The age-old myth that weight training is unsafe for children has been disproved through numerous studies. Weight training is safe for adolescents, too. The most recent population of weight trainers are octogenarians; studies of whom have proven the benefits for even the oldest among us.

Caution is recommended for all inexperienced weight trainers when learning the activity, regardless of age. That aside, most who maintain a weight training program report an increased quality of life.

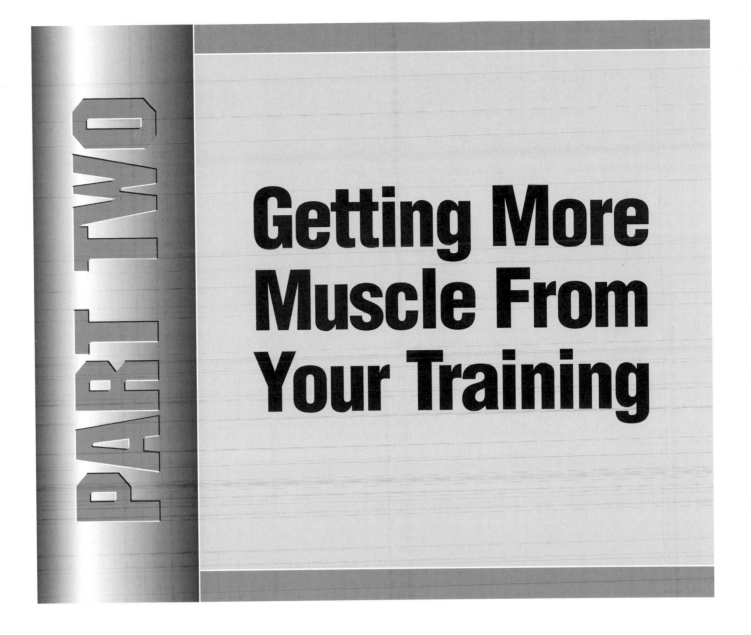

PART TWO

Getting More Muscle From Your Training

It's training time! No more general talk about how the body works. It's time for specifics. But before rushing out to grab a barbell, make sure you're clear on one very important point: *your specific training goal.*

Is your goal more *muscle mass*? More *strength and power*? More *muscular endurance*? Is your goal some combination of the above? In a goal hierarchy, are your weight training goals intended to support a higher goal (such as better sports performance)?

Why are *your specific goals* of utmost importance? There are many different weight training programs (protocols), each formulated to arrive at a different goal. Spending your time wisely requires that you follow the training path that most directly leads to fulfillment of your specific training goals.

The efficacy of matching individual goals to a particular training program can be readily seen by exploring the programs of two Olympic caliber athletes with diametrically opposite training goals, a weight lifter and a marathoner. The lifter's training goals are increased strength and power; he needs only enough cardiovascular endurance to waddle onto the lifting platform. The marathoner's training goal is expanded cardiovascular endurance; building strength and power is far down on her list of priorities.

Before reading further, study table 1, taking care to identify and appreciate the general differences distinguishing a mass program, strength and power program, and a muscular endurance program. Note that sets, reps, rest periods, exercises per body part, and training days differ for each program.

Selecting the wrong program can be more than a waste of time. The wrong program can *adversely impact* your ultimate performance. Imagine our 350-pound Olympic weight lifter running many miles every day. Imagine our marathoner with bulging muscles like Mr. Universe. It's hard to imagine without a grin, because such situations don't happen in real life—top-notch athletes are formed from a specific training mold. The concept holds true for you: Whether training to be huge, or training to look just a little better at the beach, make sure your training program is the path to your goals.

TABLE 1 Weight Training Program Comparisons

Program Elements	Strength and Power	Muscular Endurance	Muscle Mass
Exercises per muscle group	1-2	1-2	3-5
Repetitions per set	1-8	20-100	8-12
Sets per exercise	4-6	1-2	3-5
Recovery time between sets (minutes)	2½-10	1-2	½-1
Training days per week	3	3	6
Pump important?	No	No	Yes

This part of the book is divided by chapters according to three general training goals: more muscular strength and power, more muscular endurance, and more muscle mass. Which chapter is your first stop? The answer depends on a two-step process:

1. A task analysis that will lead to the desired improvement.
2. Implementing an appropriate training program.

A task analysis requires isolating the components leading to the desired improvement in performance. For example, I desire to jump higher. A task analysis indicates the muscles of the legs and hips are the primary actors in the jump. *Stronger* legs and hips will help me generate the power to jump higher.

Implementing an appropriate training program requires matching the task analysis to a specific weight training program. In my case, "*stronger* legs and hips" cues me to the training advice in chapter 6. Legs and hips would be the focus of my training. Conversely, my training time—given that my one and only goal is a higher jump—would be misspent on chapter 8, focusing on more muscle mass.

What should be the focus of *your* weight training workout? That question has as many answers as goals. If your goal is improved athletic performance in one of the scores of sports, your best bet is to solicit the advice of a coach in determining the best use of your training time regarding exercise selection. The two of you can match exercise selection and training program to the biomechanic and muscular demands of the sport.

If your goal is "merely" to develop greater strength, greater muscular endurance, or more mass, just turn to the appropriate chapter without further ado. But the primary directive still applies: narrow the focus of your workout to best meet *your* goals. Don't follow another person's program; do what's best for *you.*

The last chapter of this section describes both machine and free weight exercises that you'll need to complete your training program. The exercise descriptions are supplemented with training tips as well as a listing of the primary muscles that the exercise works.

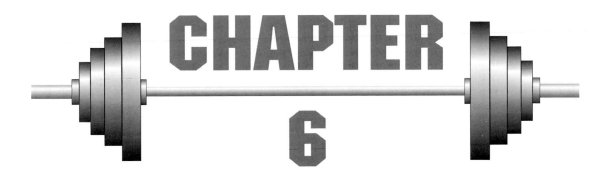

CHAPTER 6

More Muscular Strength and Power

Maybe you want to get stronger so that you can more easily tote the garbage out to the curb on Monday night. Maybe you just want to feel stronger. Whatever the reason, this is the chapter for you.

The most common reason given for strength training is improved sports performance, whether for a weekend tennis tournament or the Olympic decathlon. In fact, the overwhelming majority of successful athletes in all sports and at all levels spend many hours in a weight room, building stronger, more powerful muscles. The additional muscle is comparable to outfitting the athlete's body with state-of-the-art equipment.

Just a generation ago, weight training was anathema to most competitive sports. Typically, skill coaches feared the "muscle-bound" myth that depicted all weight trained bodies as big, slow, and inflexible. Never mind that many of their best athletes were, in fact, serious weight trainers.

Over the past two decades, increasing numbers of coaches have discovered weight training to be an indispensable training tool leading to superior performance. The burgeoning inclusion of weight training into the training regimen has dramatically impacted modern athletics. Three hundred-pound linemen capable of a 500-pound bench press—a novelty in professional football just a generation ago—are staples on today's college teams. The pendulum has swung to the point that college recruiters are as interested in a potential recruit's squat poundage as his 40-yard sprint time.

Strength training has had an equally impressive impact on females, as the narrowing gender gap in athletic performance indicates. Today's female swimmers have shattered the times recorded by males at the 1968 Olympic Games, and females have jumped higher than any male at the 1956 Olympic Games.

Whether an accomplished Olympian or a 10-year-old novice, weight training increases strength and consequent athletic performance. Those strength increases are most easily accomplished through some tried and true training methods. Let's explore.

FIRST OF ALL: WHAT IS STRENGTH?

"Strong" is a many splendored adjective in sports, and it is used in odd ways (e.g., a golfer might be said to be making a "strong charge" if she birdies a succession of holes.) It's no wonder that the distinction between muscular strength and muscular endurance is often blurred.

Designing an appropriate training program—especially choosing sets and reps—requires that the distinction between strength and muscular endurance be fully and clearly understood. A muscle's *strength*—or the strength of a group of muscles, in the case of a weight training exercise—is the greatest force the muscle can produce in a single effort. In gym terms, it's the amount of weight lifted *one* time; for example, a maximum curl, maximum squat, or maximum bench press.

The technical term for a successful best effort in a particular exercise movement is a 1 repetition maximum (1RM). Hence, a 1RM is a practical way of measuring muscular strength.

Whereas muscle strength refers to a single effort, muscle *endurance* is a measure of the muscle's ability to perform many repetitions of the same movement against a continuous resistance. For example, the number of times you could curl a 40-pound barbell would be a rough measure of your biceps' (and contributing muscles') muscular endurance.

In sports, a single, *maximum* push, heave, swing, or jump—a single maximum muscle contraction—is limited by the muscle's strength. That's the case for a discus thrower spinning his body and hurling the heavy platter, the thrust of a shot, the pull of a weightlifter, or the take-off thrust of the high jumper. On the other hand, a sprinter depends on the multiple repetitions of muscle contractions of the legs and arms churning for 50, 60, or 100 meters. Each of those multiple contractions is with less force than could be generated with a single contraction.

FINDING YOUR 1 REPETITION MAXIMUM (1RM)

For any exercise movement, finding your 1RM—the amount of weight you can lift one time—is a matter of trial and error. Start out with a bar (or very light weight), performing single lifts with a rest period in between, adding plates until the weight can no longer be lifted. For example, attempt a barbell curl with a plateless bar, and on each successive attempt add plates until the bar is too heavy to curl. The last successfully lifted weight is your 1 RM.

Few sports require only muscular strength or only muscular endurance. Nearly all require both. Brazilian soccer star Pele, who played in the U.S. professional league for several years, relied on muscular endurance to sprint the length of the field on attack and muscular strength to leap up for a head shot in front of the goal (a single, explosive effort).

The point to remember: Strength is a measure of a single, maximum effort, a single contraction of a muscle or group of muscles contributing to a movement.

STRENGTH AND POWER: THE DYNAMIC DUO

The original dynamic duo, the caped crusaders Batman and Robin, worked hand-in-hand to defeat evil forces. Strength and power, too, work as a dynamic duo to defeat opposing forces; the weight of a shot, the thrust of an opposing lineman, or the pull of gravity. A simple relationship exists between strength and power: The stronger the muscle, the more power the muscle can produce. Let's examine this fact by relating the physics of power to the biology of muscles.

Even readers who are not scientifically inclined will have little trouble with the following equation, which calculates muscle power in terms of strength and speed. Whether punching, throwing, or kicking, you can calculate muscle power as follows:

$$\text{Power} = \text{Strength (force)} \times \text{Speed.}$$

If you plug in a few numbers, you'll see that as strength increases, power increases. For example, doubling the athlete's strength—without increasing speed one iota—doubles his or her power; tripling strength triples power. Insert your own numbers into the equation to get a feel for the power potential of strength training.

The remarkable increase in power production resulting from increased strength is the underlying reason that the "power sports"—football and track and field throws (shot put, discus, hammer throw)—were the first sports to unabashedly endorse strength training. Added power, though, doesn't benefit only those athletes in traditionally defined power sports. Additional muscle power incorporates into all explosive movements. Punches, jumps, throws, and swings, a movement from nearly every sport, can be performed better with more power.

In short, a stronger athlete is a more powerful athlete and thus a better athlete.

"Quick Lifts" Build Power

As noted above, athletes and coaches in power sports were the first to climb aboard the weight training bandwagon. The so-called "quick lifts"—the clean and the snatch—quickly became the core exercises of a power-building weight training program. Why the quick lifts?

The most obvious reason is that the quick lifts require quick or "speedy" movements to hoist a heavy weight. By definition, the faster the weight is lifted through the required distance—say from floor to shoulders in the power clean—the greater the power. Power is not only required to perform the quick lifts, but also can be increased through practicing them—and power is a cherished commodity in sports.

A less obvious but equally important reason to include quick lifts in a sports workout is this: Quick lifts emphasize the body's major muscle groups in the same sequence as the typical power event. That point can be better understood by comparing the primary muscular emphasis at different stages of the power clean and shot put.

Both the power clean and the shot put depend on the same sequence of muscular emphasis: leg drive, hip thrust, torso flexion, shoulder thrust, and finally arm drive. In fact, that same sequence of muscular action—leg-hip-torso-shoulder-arm—the so-called "power train," holds true for a lineman's thrust, a boxer's punch, a quarterback's throw, a rower's pull, and for most other sporting events as well.

No exercises are better at sequencing that power train than the quick lifts. As the muscles involved in the power train sequence become stronger and learn to work in tandem, the body's overall power output increases. And athletic performance improves. A generic quick lift program is included at the end of this chapter.

Myth: Those Big, Slow Weight Lifters

Myth: Weight training hurts the athlete's speed, turning him or her into a slow, immobile blob of useless muscle. Fact: Weight training usually increases the athlete's speed.

Greater muscular strength more easily overcomes external resistance; this is the mechanism of improved speed. Imagine a 100-meter sprinter; knees driving, arms pumping, exploding forward with each step. Now imagine him twice as strong, each muscle more powerful than before. Those stronger muscles help him overcome the force of gravity, increasing stride length and frequency. In fact, that's why the vast majority of world-class sprinters spend a substantial portion of total training time in a weight room.

STICK TO SPECIFICS

If you *strength* train to improve athletic performance, your weight room exercises should duplicate your sport's movements as closely as possible. The closer the training exercise matches the speed, motion, and resistance of competition, the more likely the increased muscular power built through weight training will contribute to the power of the competition movement.

Whatever the event, stronger muscles breed faster movements. However, keep in mind that speed, like strength, is highly specific. Practically speaking, that means you must strengthen the muscles involved in an athletic movement to increase the speed of that movement. In other words, bench pressing won't build faster legs, but squatting will.

The important point is that each muscle and every derivative athletic movement can be strengthened. Increased muscle strength will bring faster movements.

SETS, REPS, WEIGHT, AND TRAINING DAYS

How many sets, reps, weights, and training days are most effective in building strength? Believe it or not, that's one of the most controversial questions in weight training, because what's *best* for the individual weight trainer depends on a compilation of age, maturity, other activities, training intensity, motivation, specific genetic gifts, and personality.

Statistically, *three sets of six repetitions* (not counting warm-up sets), *three workouts per week*, is the typical, strength-building set-rep pattern for experienced weight trainers. The ambiguous words "statistically" and "typical" are necessary in the foregoing statement on sets and reps because no one set-rep-rest pattern fits all people. The basis of analysis for the three-six-three pattern is analogous to the "average" heights and weights routinely used to represent the diversity of humanity.

Six sets of six reps, three days per week, have been shown to accomplish a greater rate of strength increase, if the athlete has the additional time, recuperative powers, and energy to spend in the gym.

Statistics are based on averages, and averages cloud the most interesting cases. For example, Kirk Karwoski, world power lifting record holder for the three-lift total with a 970-pound squat, 560-pound bench, and 820-pound deadlift, is a 280-pounder who trains each body part *once* a week. He divides the body into legs, back, and upper body. That's three workouts per week, one for each body part. For example, that means squats once each week. His typical workout: after warm-up sets, *one all-out, five-rep set.*

Olympic weight lifters, demonstrably the most powerful people in sports, frequently train with a system first popularized by the Bulgarian weight lifting team. The lifter trains six days per week, three times per day (18 workouts per week). Each workout consists of three exercises— snatch, clean and jerk, and squat. After a warm-up, the athlete performs six single repetitions of each exercise movement. Each repetition is with a 100% maximum weight. That's 18 maximum repetitions per workout, three workouts per day, six days per week, a total of 324 maximum lifts per week. It works for them.

Finding what will work best for you is a matter of trial and error. In the meantime, consider the recommendations listed on the workout charts found in the following section. They will build strength even if they are not perfectly matched to your particular physical and psychological profile. Don't be afraid to experiment, though—within the parameters of age and experience—to find an individualized training sequence that best suits your individual needs and abilities.

PROFILE: CHRIS SPRAGUE

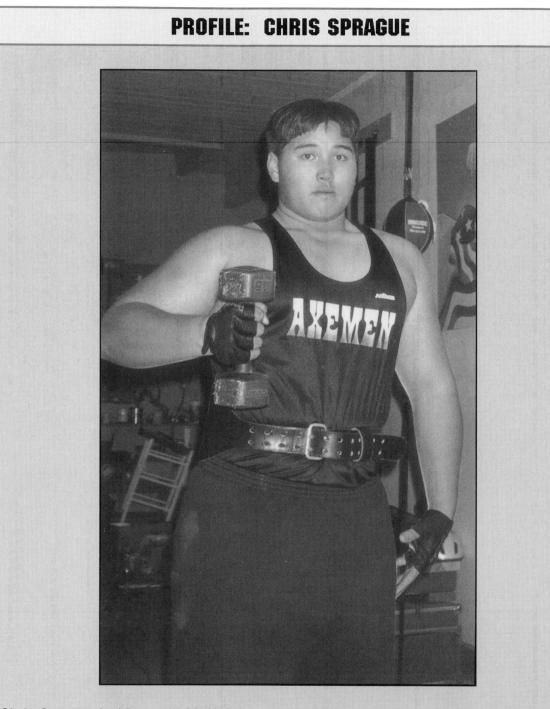

Chris Sprague is 15 years old. He's strong. And wide! Although well within the normal range for height at a little over six feet tall, he carries 290 pounds with 20-inch arms and 35-inch thighs that already full squat with over 600 pounds.

Chris started weight training as a 10-year-old, wanting to join his father on a "fun" trip to the gym. Soon thereafter, weight training became a vehicle that Chris rode to improved sports performance. Chris has won five National Junior Olympic Track and Field Championships with the stronger, bigger, quicker body he built through weight training.

Chris' primary weight training goal is strength. He trains all year, even during football and track seasons. Less time is spent in the weight room during the sports seasons, but every training day is an all-out effort. The following program (not for the faint-of-heart) is how Chris has made truly incredible gains. Keep in mind, however, that Chris trained for four years before having the power base for such an intense workout.

One important note: "Maximum intensity" means that Chris uses a weight that, on his own, he could lift one or two repetitions. He does the one or two reps and is then helped through an additional five repetitions by his training partner. That's a total of six or seven repetitions per "maximum set" (one or two alone, five with help). The rationale for this training method is that each of the six or seven repetitions is at or near maximum overload.

Some exercises can't be safely performed with a helper; for example, a power clean. Imagine having four hands on the bar during a power clean. For those exercises, the traditional set-rep combinations are listed.

MAXIMUM INTENSITY STRENGTH PROGRAM

Muscle group	Exercise	Sets	Reps	Days/week
Quadriceps	Squats	3	Maximum intensity	M/Th
	Leg Press (single-leg)	2	Maximum intensity	M/Th
	Lunge	2	8	M/Th
Pectorals	Incline Press	3	Maximum intensity	Tu/Sa
	Seated Bench Press (isolateral single-arm)	3	Maximum intensity	Tu/Sa
	Fly Machine	3	Maximum intensity	Tu/Sa
Deltoids	Dumbbell Shoulder Press	4	8-6-6-6	Tu/Sa
Trapezius, erector spinae	Power Clean	5	6-3-3-3-1	Tu/Sa
	Deadlift	4	6-3-3-1	Once a week (following Power Clean)
Abdominals	Sit-Ups	2	Maximum intensity	Tu/Sa

STRENGTH AND POWER TRAINING PROGRAMS

There are two basic strength- and power-building programs. Each of the programs embodies the same goals: building strength and power in the athlete's major muscle groups. The programs' differences reflect exercise and intensity adjustments dependent on the experience of the athlete.

The choice of the word athlete is not arbitrary. The fact is that the majority of people focusing on building strength and power—as opposed to pure muscle mass and shape—are athletes seeking improved athletic performance. If athletic improvement is your goal, the Sport-Specific Strength and Power Training Programs at the end of this chapter are for you.

The fact that athletes wanting to improve athletic performance comprise the largest segment of strength trainers isn't meant to exclude those of you wanting more strength for other reasons; perhaps to open a jar of jelly more easily or increase a sense of competence in performing everyday physical activities.

All the exercises found in this book will build strength, but not *all* of them can be included in one or two strength training programs. Hence, the following Muscle Strength and Power Training Programs represent a manageable, effective group of exercises guaranteed to increase the athlete's overall strength/power base—and the power base of the nonathlete, too.

Why aren't traditionally popular exercises like triceps extensions included in the programs? For a clear explanation, let's compare the squat, an exercise movement included in the program, to the triceps extension.

SELECTING A WEIGHT FOR MUSCLE STRENGTH AND POWER WORKOUT PROGRAM

The rule of thumb: Selecting a weight is a matter of trial and error over several workouts because we all have different strength levels. For each exercise, every individual requires a different weight for his or her six to eight repetitions.

If you're a beginner, select your proper weight for each exercise as follows:

◆ With all leg and back exercises, start the experimentation with 25% of your body weight when using both arms and legs.

◆ With all leg and back exercises, start the experimentation with 20% of your body weight when using single-arm or single-leg movements.

◆ Begin with no added resistance (no weight) when starting abdominal exercises.

This approach will help you decide if you've selected too heavy or too light a weight so you can adjust accordingly over your next several workouts. In several weeks of workouts, you will find what your correct load is for each lift. Caveat—it's better to select too light a weight than too heavy when experimenting to find your correct load.

The squatting movement requires intense work of the large muscles of the thighs, hips, back, and abdominals—that's more than 50% of your body's total muscle mass. On the other hand, the triceps extension requires only some of the muscles of the arm; at most, 10% of your body's total muscle mass. Hence, increasing the strength and power of muscles responsible for the squatting movement would add more overall power than an equivalent percentage strength increase of the muscles responsible for the triceps extension. Furthermore, the triceps are effectively worked by other exercise movements (i.e., bench press) that are included in the strength and power program.

You may still want to include the triceps extension in your power building routine, but you'll get the most power for your buck with the recommended exercises in the muscle strength and power workouts at the end of this chapter. Why the adjustments for experience? The primary reason is safety. For example, overhead lifts are much more appropriate (that is, safe) for an experienced weight trainer. The reason for excluding overhead lifts goes beyond the prospect of a barbell colliding with a skull. Muscle injuries (especially back and shoulder) are more common for an inexperienced lifter attempting overhead lifts. Hence, overhead lifts are excluded from the basic program.

Why have kids and beginners been grouped under the same program? Kids usually lack weight training experience, and they can't be expected to conform to the same standards of gym conduct (i.e., safety practices) as adults. There's one more reason: The American Pediatric Association officially recommends that kids not perform overhead lifts. That recommendation is also based on safety considerations (as discussed in chapter 5).

There are kids who can safely follow the same program as an adult. However, these kids represent the exception, not the rule. Kids who have been lifting for several years under expert supervision, and are still supervised by qualified adults, are also the exception.

Use the Quick Lifts Program, the Muscle Strength and Power Training Programs, or the Sport-Specific Strength and Power Training Programs that follow to help you achieve your strength goals.

QUICK LIFTS PROGRAM

Muscle group	Exercise	Sets	Reps	Days/week
Quadriceps	Squat	5	6	M/Th
All muscle groups	Power Clean	5	6	M/Th
Abdominals	Sit-Ups	2	10	M/Th

Note. The squat, not a quick lift, is included as part of the program to incorporate the all-important power base of the legs, which is essential to mastering quick lifts.

Tu/F, W/Sa, and Th/Su are acceptable substitutes for training days.

MUSCLE STRENGTH AND POWER TRAINING PROGRAMS

BASIC PROGRAM

Muscle group	Exercise	Sets	Reps	Days/ week	Page no.
Quadriceps	Leg Press	3	8	M/Th	106
	Step-Ups	3	8	M/Th	112
Pectorals	Bench Press	5	6-8	M/Th	126-133
Erector spinae	Back Extension	3	8	M/Th	154
Latissimus dorsi	Pull-Ups	5	6	M/Th	150
Trapezius	Shoulder Shrugs	3	8	M/Th	146-149
Abdominals	Sit-Ups	3	8	M/Th	194

ADVANCED PROGRAM

Muscle group	Exercise	Sets	Reps	Days/ week	Page no.
Quadriceps	Squat	5	6	M/Th	108
	Lunge	3	8	M	110
	Leg Press	3	8	M	106
Pectorals	Bench Press	5	6	M	126-133
Deltoids	Push Press	5	6	Th	162-165
Trapezius, erector spinae	Power Clean[a]	3	6	Th	142
	Deadlift	5	3-6	Th	144
Abdominals	Sit-Ups	3	8	Th	194

Note. *Tu/F, W/Sa, and Th/Su are acceptable substitutes for training days. The point is to space the training days to allow for maximum rest.*

The set and rep recommendations do not include warm-up sets. Two warm-up sets are recommended, the first at 25% of 1RM, and a second at 50% of 1RM.

[a]*Perform the Power Clean before the Deadlift. The converse order—deadlift before power clean— would exhaust the lower back, preventing the explosiveness necessary for effectively executing power cleans.*

SPORT-SPECIFIC STRENGTH AND POWER TRAINING PROGRAMS

BASEBALL-SOFTBALL

Muscle group	Exercise	Sets	Reps	Days/ week	Page no.
Quadriceps	Squat	5	8	M/F	108
	Lunge	2	8	M/W/F	110
Hip flexors, abdominals	Knee-Ups	3	8	M/W/F	198
	Reverse Trunk Twist	2	12	M/W/F	196
Trapezius, erector spinae	Power Clean	5	6	W	142
	Deadlift	5	6-8	M/W/F	144
Deltoids, triceps	Machine Push Press	3	8	M/W/F	164

BASKETBALL

Muscle group	Exercise	Sets	Reps	Days/ week	Page no.
Quadriceps	Squat or Leg Press	5	6-8	M/F	108, 106
	Lunge	3	8	M/W/F	110
Pectorals, triceps	Bench Press (close grip)	3	8	M/W/F	126-133
Latissimus dorsi, biceps	Machine Pull-Down (close grip)	3	8	M/W/F	152
Trapezius, erector spinae	Deadlift	3	8	W	144
Abdominals, hip flexors	Knee-Ups	3	10	M/W/F	198
Calves	Machine Calf Raise	3	10-12	M/W/F	122-125

BOXING

Muscle group	Exercise	Sets	Reps	Days/ week	Page no.
Quadriceps	Lunge	3	8	M/W/F	110
	Step-Ups	2	8	W	112
	Leg Press	5	8	M/F	106
Pectorals	Barbell Bench Press	3	8	M/W/F	126
Abdominals	Sit-Ups	3	8	M/W/F	194
	Reverse Trunk Twist	5	10	M/W/F	196
Deltoids	Alternating Upright Row	2	8	M/W/F	170
Trapezius, erector spinae	Deadlift	6	20[a]	M/W/F	144

FOOTBALL (LINEMAN)

Muscle group	Exercise	Sets	Reps	Days/ week	Page no.
Quadriceps	Squat	6	6	M/F	108
	Lunge	3	8	M/W/F	110
Trapezius, erector spinae	Power Clean	5	6	M/W/F	142
	Deadlift	5	5-8	M/F	144
Deltoids	Push Press	3	8	M/W/F	162-165
Abdominals	Sit-Ups	3	8	M/W/F	194
	Reverse Trunk Twist	3	8	M/W/F	196

GOLF

Muscle group	Exercise	Sets	Reps	Days/ week	Page no.
Quadriceps	Step-Ups	2	8	M/W/F	112
	Lunge	3	8	M/F	110
Deltoids	Alternating Upright Row	3	8	M/W/F	170
Trapezius, erector spinae	Deadlift	5	8	W	144
Latissimus dorsi, biceps	Pull-Ups	3	8	M/W/F	150
Abdominals	Sit-Ups	3	8	M/W/F	194

[a]*Muscle endurance/overall power activity*

MARTIAL ARTS

Muscle group	Exercise	Sets	Reps	Days/week	Page no.
Quadriceps	Lunge	5	8	M/W/F	110
	Squat	5	6-8	M/F	108
Trapezius, erector spinae	Power Clean	3	8	M/W/F	142
	Deadlift	3	8	M/F	144
Deltoids	Push Press	3	8	M/W/F	162-165
Abdominals	Sit-Ups	3	8	M/W/F	194
	Reverse Trunk Twist	5	8	M/W/F	196

SHOT PUT, DISCUS, AND HAMMER

Muscle group	Exercise	Sets	Reps	Days/week	Page no.
Quadriceps	Squat	6	6	M/F	108
	Leg Press	4	8	M/F	106
Abdominals	Sit-Ups	3	10	M/W/F	194
	Reverse Trunk Twist	3	10	M/W/F	196
Trapezius, erector spinae	Power Clean	5	6	W	142
	Deadlift	5	5	W	144
Pectorals	Bench Press	6	6	M/F	126-133

VOLLEYBALL

Muscle group	Exercise	Sets	Reps	Days/week	Page no.
Quadriceps	Squat	4	8	M/W/F	108
	Lunge	4	10	M/W/F	110
Latissimus dorsi	Machine Pull-Down	3	8	M/W/F	152
Pectorals	Bench Press	4	8-10	M/W/F	126-133
Calves	Machine Calf Raise	4	12	M/F	122-125
Abdominals, hip flexors	Knee-Ups	5	10	M/W/F	198
Trapezius, erector spinae	Deadlift	3	10	M/F	144
Deltoids	Alternating Upright Row	4	8	M/W/F	170

CLOSING SET

As noted earlier, all the exercises found in this book will build strength and power. The exercises selected for the programs in this chapter were chosen because they provide a total body workout that, rep per rep, incorporates the most muscle.

Selection of an appropriate combination of sets, reps, and training days is crucial to a successful strength and power program. Statistically, three sets of six repetitions, three days per week, are typical training protocols for the experienced weight trainer. However, the "best" training protocol is highly individualistic and is best arrived at through trial and error—always proceeding cautiously and avoiding overtraining in the process.

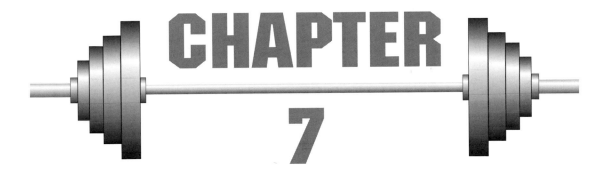

CHAPTER 7

More Muscular Endurance

The starter's pistol sounds. Carl Lewis bursts from the starting blocks and sprints 100 meters to the tape, arms and legs pumping furiously all the way. Mike Tyson stands in the middle of the ring and slugs it out with his opponent, each of them throwing combinations of punches so rapid that the ringside broadcaster gets tongue-tied. Lee Haney, eight-time Mr. Olympia, repeatedly curls a heavy barbell, rep after grueling rep. And Gwen Torrance sprints to a victory in the 100 meters at the World Championships. These are examples of *anaerobic* or *muscular-endurance* activities—activities requiring such a rapid succession of near maximal muscle contractions that energy is used faster than the bloodstream can supply oxygen to produce it.

Anaerobic events in sports typically are those involving repeated, near-maximal muscular contractions lasting from five seconds through one or two minutes. That time frame readily encompasses the typical bodybuilding set.

Muscular-endurance or anaerobic events differ from muscular-strength events (e.g., the shot put, or a single, maximum lift), which require one explosive muscular contraction at a time, and from aerobic or cardiovascular-endurance events (e.g., the marathon), which rely on the heart and bloodstream for a continuous supply of oxygen to fuel countless repetitions of muscle contractions. Hence, a muscle's endurance comes into play somewhere between one and countless muscular contractions.

Muscular endurance (anaerobic endurance)—whether during a set of curls or a 100-meter dash—relies on its own fuel system, the energy-producing deposits of glycogen (carbohydrates) stored within the muscle cell. However, these stored deposits can produce only a limited supply of energy. After one to two minutes of repeated, intense contractions, the muscle can no longer rely on the glycogen stores for energy. At that moment, Lewis, Tyson, Haney,

Torrance, or any other athlete feels exhaustion and pain, and the ability to produce rapid, near maximal muscular contractions is lost.

NO PAIN, NO GAIN?

Have you ever wondered why "no pain, no gain" has become the weight trainer's battle cry? It's because rapid, intense muscle contractions create a "burning" sensation, a sensation the early weight trainers described as painful. The burn is a product of the weight trainer's reliance on the anaerobic energy system, the energy system that draws on energy stored within the muscle, in an energy emergency. Although pain is traditionally viewed as the body's way of communicating distress or injury, the painful burning sensation brought about by the rapid, intense muscle contractions is a sought-after prize by hard-core bodybuilders. Schwarzenegger, hard-core bodybuilder extraordinaire, put this painful burn in its place: "If you can make it through the pain period, you can make it to be a champion. And if you can't go through, forget it." Most of us "forget it" and accept more modest muscular development.

Earlier, we saw that two wholly different energy production pathways—the aerobic (with oxygen) and anaerobic (without oxygen) systems—independently operate to provide the energy requirements for all of the athlete's muscle contractions. Which system provides the bulk of energy at any given time depends on the rate and intensity of muscular contractions.

The aerobic system marvelously hums along around the clock, providing energy for routine, ongoing, low-intensity muscular contractions, such as those required to turn the pages of this book, propel the breathing apparatus throughout the day, or power the legs during a long walk through the woods. The aerobic system relies on an ongoing delivery of oxygen to your muscle cells, wherein that oxygen produces energy through chemical reactions. You're unaware of the continuous aerobic chemical reactions taking place within your muscle cells. The oxygen-carbohydrate reactions efficiently and painlessly produce energy for low-intensity muscle contractions, and the waste products of these oxygen-carbohydrate reactions are just as efficiently and painlessly carried away from the muscle cell by the ever present stream of blood.

What happens, then, in a muscular emergency demanding a continuous production of *high-intensity*, near maximal, muscular contractions requiring more energy than is available through the oxygen-carbohydrate (aerobic) reactions? For example, the apartment catches fire, and you have to run down five flights of stairs to escape the flames. Or when you sprint 200 yards at the end of a long race? Or when you force your legs to endure 20 reps of a heavy squat?

Rapid, high-intensity, near maximal muscular contractions (e.g., the contractions of a 20-rep set of squats) hit the body like an emergency and call into play an emergency energy system, the anaerobic system. The anaerobic system arrives at the emergency with its own set of energy-producing rules.

The first rule of the anaerobic energy system is to produce energy *without* oxygen. The rule is dictated by the urgency of the emergency: Oxygen reactions would take too long to produce enough energy necessary to recharge high-intensity muscle contractions. The bloodstream can't deliver oxygen fast enough to fuel the oxygen-carbohydrate reaction. Hence, the anaerobic system orchestrates short-term chemical reactions that release energy from carbohydrates without oxygen.

There is a price to this shortcut in energy production to meet the muscular emergency. The burning sensation is produced by lactic acid, an end product of the oxygen-depleted chemical reactions. Pain is the signal that too much lactic acid has accumulated in the muscle cell; it can't take much more stress.

On a positive note, this burning sensation (not the sharp pain signaling an injury) can be interpreted by the athlete as a signal that the high-rep activity e.g., a 20- rep set of squats or a 200-meter sprint) has successfully overloaded the working muscle. In other words, the short-term burning sensation produced by anaerobic training produces long-term gains.

Have you ever put forth a quick burst of energy—running up the stairs, chasing your dog, or running the bases at the company picnic—that's left you exhausted, with an almost sick feeling? The chances are that the awful feeling is attributable to the lactic acid that accumulates in the temporarily overworked muscle cell from the repeated, high-intensity muscle contractions. The lactic acid must be removed before the muscle cell can perform another intense set of contractions.

Ironically, oxygen is required to rid the cell of the lactic acid. An oxygen reaction transforms the toxic lactic acid into benign chemical compounds. That's why you pant and gasp for air *after* you have completed the unexpectedly intense activity. The panting continues until enough oxygen, via the bloodstream, breaks down the lactic acid and hauls away the harmless byproducts. In other words, the panting continues until you have repaid the "oxygen debt" owed those tired, overworked muscles.

THE CONNECTION BETWEEN STRENGTH AND MUSCULAR ENDURANCE

Earlier, we outlined the *distinction* between muscular strength and muscular endurance—strength is the measure of one maximum muscle contraction; muscular endurance (anaerobic power) is the measure of numerous contractions against a fixed resistance. Now let's state the *connection* between strength and muscular endurance: Assuming that all other conditioning factors are equal, the stronger athlete has greater muscular endurance.

Hurdler Edwin Moses, or rowers on the Harvard crew, can use a smaller proportion of their total strength (and thus less effort) to create the same thrust as their weaker opponents. In other words, movement after movement, they operate far less near their maximal capacity than their weaker opponents to produce the same thrust of leg or oar. This leaves more fuel in the muscular tank for the stronger athletes, so they run out of gas less quickly.

For another example, let's say Bob can manage to do a single squatting movement with 600 pounds, while Joe can squat once with 300 pounds. Both men have followed the same training program of sets and reps except that Bob uses heavier weights, reflecting his superior strength. If both men test their muscular endurance by squatting with a bar on their shoulders weighing 200 pounds, Bob will be able to perform more squats than Joe. The strength has, in effect, given Bob a muscular endurance (anaerobic power) advantage when squatting. Of course, muscular endurance is highly specific: Joe may be able to outperform Bob in all other movements.

The strength-muscular endurance connection is one of the reasons males have an advantage over females in athletic competitions that depend on muscular endurance. Because males can develop greater strength, it follows that they can achieve greater muscular endurance (more repetitions per unit time) against an equivalent resistance (cardiovascular endurance is another matter altogether).

To prove the connection we're referring to, find a friend who is substantially stronger or weaker than you are. Using a bag of potatoes, sugar, or other weights, begin lifting. The weight should be approximately half the maximum single-lift capacity of the weaker person. Both of you should curl the weights in rapid cadence. Which of you can curl the weight more times? The stronger person

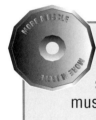

Bodybuilding, because of the intense sets of 8 to 15 repetitions executed within 15 to 30 seconds, is technically within the scope of a muscular endurance activity.

has the greater muscular endurance—assuming that neither of you have been practicing lifting sacks of sugar or potatoes.

STICK TO SPECIFICS

If you're weight training to improve athletic performance, your weight room exercises should duplicate your sport's movements as closely as possible. The closer the training exercise matches the speed, motion, and resistance of competition, the more probable the increased muscular endurance built during training will apply during competition. The following anecdote will help clarify the concept.

John Greenshields, a 28-year-old FBI agent, did 14,000 sit-ups in a row at the Tampa, Florida, YMCA in 1964. The feat took him 6 hours, 10 minutes. He had practiced by doing 1,000 sit-ups before breakfast every day, another 500 before going to bed, and even more on weekends. Quite a feat—but he was preparing to set a record, period.

Specificity in muscular endurance training simply means that the athlete should use the muscles during training as they will be used during competition. Just as important, the training speed, strength, and technique should match the hoped-for competition speed, strength, and technique. If Greenshields was doing all those sit-ups in preparation for a marathon, his training time was wasted. He should have been working on his legs and cardiovascular system.

A common waste of training time when preparing for an anaerobic event is jogging, an activity which doesn't prepare the athlete for the same muscular endurance demands of competition. How many times during a boxing match does a boxer jog? Never; his leg movements need to be much more explosive and rapidly sequenced than the humdrum rhythm of jogging. Jogging is good only for general cardiovascular conditioning, not for muscular endurance—unless the level of muscular endurance sought is that demanded of jogging.

For an example of the right way to train using specificity, consider a runner preparing to run 800 meters in 2 minutes in competition. During training, he runs 400 meters in 60 seconds or less, 200 meters in 30 seconds or less, and 100 meters in 15 seconds or less. You can see that each distance is covered at the same pace as that planned for the race, or faster. The muscular demands on the athlete during training match the demands of the race; thus, he or she will be prepared. The principle of specificity holds for weight training exercises, too: You're going to increase muscular endurance only in those muscles that you exercise. In other words, the muscular endurance (anaerobic power) of the legs won't increase one iota from hundreds of sets of curls.

In fact, the principle of specificity holds true whether the event be the 800-meter run, boxing, tennis, or any other muscular endurance activity. In short: Train for muscular endurance exactly as you expect to compete.

PROFILE: PAULA SCHAFFER

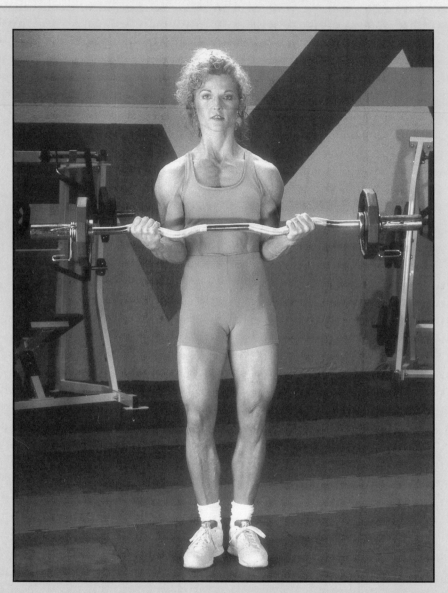

Paula Schaffer won the Master's Natural Bodybuilding Competition in March 1995. This 40+-year-old athlete is happily married to Steve Schaffer, has four children, and works as a personal trainer.

Paula keeps a journal of what she does, how she trains, and what she eats—trying to make a science of bodybuilding. Nevertheless, success takes more than science—it takes work, too: "Getting lean is hard. The truth hurts: becoming successful in bodybuilding means lots of suffering and sacrifice to lose weight. I follow a nearly vegetarian diet. In short, it takes two things to compete: one, a positive mental approach; and two, proper nutrition."

Here's Paula's overview of her workout, which develops a combination of strength and muscular endurance: "I lift only two days per week. Everything is done one set to failure. Some sets are done with a breakdown to protect my low back. I use primarily Hammer Strength machines at my gym."

FIRST WEEKLY WORKOUT PROGRAM

Muscle group	Exercise	Weight	Reps	Breakdown reps
Hamstrings	Seated Leg Curl	7-8		12
Quadriceps	Leg Press (seat close up, no rest between)	300 lb	5-6	8-10
	Squat (slow)	None	6 (10 seconds down; 10 seconds up)	
Deltoids, trapezius	Machine Upright Row	Heavy	6	5-6
	Shoulder Shrug Machine	Heavy	6	5-6
Latissimus dorsi	Single Arm Pull-Downs	Heavy	5	8
Triceps	Lying Barbell Extension	45 lb	10-12	6-8
Calves	Seated Calf Machine	Heavy	10	10
Abdominals	Abdominal Crunches	None	30 (with 4-second hold in contracted state)	
	Oblique Crunches or Knee Raises	None	25-30	

SECOND WEEKLY WORKOUT PROGRAM

Muscle group	Exercise	Weight	Reps	Breakdown reps
Quadriceps	Leg Extension Machine	Heavy	8-9	5-7
	Leg Press Machine (with low foot position at 45°, toes out)	Heavy	6-8	10-12
	Step-Ups		10-12	
Pectorals	10° Fly Machine	Heavy	8-10	
	Wide Chest Machine	Heavy	8-10	
Deltoids	Lateral Raise Machine	Heavy	8-10	
Biceps	Barbell Curls		10-14	
	Biceps Curl Machine		10-12	
Calves	Seated Calf Machine		15-20	
Abdominals	Abdominal Crunches		30 (with 4-second hold in contracted state)	
	Oblique Crunches or Knee Raises		25-30	

Note. Breakdown reps are assisted reps that follow the initial rep count. In Paula's case, her training partner removes weight from the bar as she fatigues.

MUSCULAR ENDURANCE TRAINING PROGRAMS

Years of experimentation with various training methods have shown that the best system for developing muscular endurance is interval training: alternate periods of intense anaerobic exercise (work intervals) and rest periods (muscle recovery intervals) in a workout. That's the case for sprinting, boxing, and the traditional weight training workout!

The work intervals are short periods of intense, all-out exertions at 90 to 100% capacity. They are necessarily short, as it is impossible to move at or near 100% capacity for longer than very brief periods (one to two minutes). And the intensity of the exercise must be at least 90% of maximum; any less effort, and you can't count on the muscles to adapt with greater muscular endurance.

It's easy to figure the magical, 90% level of training intensity for sports that are timed and measured, such as swimming and track and field—just calculate 90% of the athlete's best effort. For example, the 400-meter runner capable of a one-minute race will run 360 meters during a one-minute work interval (90% of 400 meters is 360 meters).

The same rough calculations can be used to determine 90% intensity in a weight training exercise. If, on his best day, the athlete can curl 10 reps with a 100-pound barbell, a 9-rep set with the same weight (100 pounds) meets the magical 90% level. The same method of calculation holds true for sets of greater repetitions. If, on her best day, the athlete can perform a given number of reps—20, 30, or 50—with a given weight, performing 90% of that rep count on a normal training day is a great workout.

With high-intensity, muscular endurance training, a balance must exist between work and recovery intervals. Recovery must be long enough to allow the muscles to eliminate the accumulated lactic acid. As you might expect, a longer work interval demands a longer recovery interval. A 15-second work interval (10-12 exercise reps) might require two minutes of recovery, whereas a 2-minute work interval (60-80 exercise reps) might necessitate a recovery interval of 15 minutes. The longer the work interval, the longer the time needed to eliminate the lactic acid and replenish the energy network. A generic muscular endurance model is outlined in table 7.1.

TABLE 7.1 GENERIC MUSCULAR ENDURANCE WORKOUT MODEL

Exercises per muscle group	2
Repetitions per set	30
Sets per exercise	2
Recovery time between sets	2 minutes
Training days per week	3—Monday, Wednesday, Friday

Although studies are inconclusive, it appears that interval training sessions—regardless of sport—should be practiced every other day. (Keep in mind that we are training for muscular endurance, not cardiovascular endurance.) Not coincidentally, that's the traditional weight training regimen: one day of training followed by one day of rest.

With all of the above in mind, the Basic Muscular Endurance Training Program at the end of this chapter provides a sample workout program to improve muscular endurance. This is the workout for you if your goal is generalized improvement in muscular endurance. Remember, though, that like Greenshields and his sit-ups, you're building muscular endurance *only* in the muscles incorporated in the exercise routine.

You needn't limit your options when selecting muscular endurance exercises. If you're weight training for improved sports performance, the most important consideration in your exercise selection is to match the exercise movement as closely as possible to the sporting movement. Check out the Sport-Specific Endurance Training Programs in this chapter for some sample workouts.

SELECTING A WEIGHT: LOW WEIGHTS FOR HIGH REPS

The rule of thumb: Selecting a weight is a matter of trial and error over several workouts because we all have different muscular endurance levels. For each exercise, every individual requires a different weight for his or her 25 repetitions.

If you're a beginner, select your proper weight for each exercise as follows:

◆ With all leg and back exercises, start the experimentation with 10% of your body weight when using both arms and legs.

◆ When using one arm or leg in a lift, even though it seems extremely light, begin the experimentation with 5% of your body weight.

◆ Begin with no added resistance (no weight) when starting the knee-ups (abdominal) exercises.

This approach will help you decide if the weight you've selected is too heavy or too light, and you can adjust accordingly over your next several workouts. In several weeks of workouts, you will find what your correct load is for each lift. Caveat—It's better to select too light a weight than too heavy when experimenting to find your correct load.

BASIC MUSCULAR ENDURANCE TRAINING PROGRAM

Muscle group	Exercise	Sets	Reps	Days/week	Page no.
Quadriceps	Lunge (Dumbbell)	1-2	25	M/W/F	110
	Lunge (Barbell)	1-2	25	M/W/F	110
	Step-Ups	1-2	25	M/W/F	112
Abdominals	Knee-Ups	1-2	25	M/W/F	198
Erector spinae	Back Extension	1-2	25	M/W/F	154
Trapezius, erector spinae	Deadlift	1-2	25	M/W/F	144
Pectorals	Bench Press	1-2	25	M/W/F	126-133
Latissimus dorsi	Machine Pull-Down	1-2	25	M/W/F	152

These set and rep recommendations do not include warm-up sets.

One warm-up set is recommended: Use 20% of your 1RM.

Sets: Begin by performing one set of all exercises. As muscular endurance and training capacity increase over time, move to two sets per exercise.

Rest Periods: Quickly move from set to set, from exercise to exercise, minimizing as much as possible the rest period between sets. Over time, the rest periods will decrease as the body learns to adapt to the lactic acid buildup in the blood.

SPORT-SPECIFIC ENDURANCE TRAINING PROGRAMS

CYCLING

Muscle group	Exercise	Sets	Reps	Days/week	Page no.
Quadriceps	Step-Ups	3	25	M/W/F	112
	Leg Press	2	20	M/W/F	106
Hamstrings	Leg Curl	2	50	M/W/F	114-117
Trapezius, erector spinae	Power Clean	2	25	M/W/F	142
	Deadlift	1	20	M/W/F	144
Abdominals	Knee-Ups	2	50	M/W/F	198
	Reverse Trunk Twist	1	50	M/W/F	196
Deltoids	Alternating Upright Row	2	20	M/W/F	170
Triceps, pectorals, deltoids	Dip	2	20	M/W/F	134
Latissimus dorsi, biceps, erector spinae	Seated Long Pull	2	30	M/W/F	160

ROWING

Muscle group	Exercise	Sets	Reps	Days/week	Page no.
Quadriceps	Leg Press	2	20	M/F	106
Trapezius, erector spinae	Power Clean	2	20	M/F	142
	Deadlift	1	20	M/F	144
Abdominals	Sit-Ups	1	40	M/F	194
Latissimus dorsi, biceps, erector spinae	Seated Long Pull	3	30	M/F	160

SKIING

Muscle group	Exercise	Sets	Reps	Days/week	Page no.
Quadriceps	Leg Press	2	20	M/F	106
	Squat	2	20	M/F	108
	Lunge	2	20	M/F	110
Trapezius, erector spinae	Power Clean	2	20	M/F	142
	Bench Press (close grip)	3	10-12	M/W/F	126-133
Erector spinae	Back Extension	2	20	M/W/F	154
Abdominals	Sit-Ups	1	40	M/W/F	194
Latissimus dorsi, biceps, erector spinae	Seated Long Pull	2	20	M/W/F	160
Hamstrings	Leg Curl	2	15	M/W/F	114-117

SOCCER

Muscle group	Exercise	Sets	Reps	Days/week	Page no.
Quadriceps	Squat	2	20	M/F	108
	Lunge	2	30	W	110
Trapezius, erector spinae	Deadlift	2	20	M/F	144
Latissimus dorsi, biceps	Pull-Ups	2	Maximum	M/F	150
Hamstrings	Leg Curl	2	20	M/F	114-117
Abdominals, hip flexors	Knee-Ups	3	10	M/W/F	198

SPRINTS

Muscle group	Exercise	Sets	Reps	Days/ week	Page no.
Quadriceps	Step-Ups	2	30	M/W/F	112
	Lunge	2	20	M/W/F	110
Abdominals	Reverse Trunk Twist	1	30	M/W/F	196
Hip Flexors	Knee-Ups	2	30	M/W/F	198
Hamstrings	Leg Curl	2	20	M/W/F	114-117
Trapezius, erector spinae	Power Clean	2	20	M/W/F	142
Latissimus dorsi, biceps, erector spinae	Seated Long Pull	1	25	M/W/F	160

SWIMMING

Muscle group	Exercise	Sets	Reps	Days/ week	Page no.
Abdominals	Sit-Ups	2	25	M/F	194
Erector spinae	Back Extension	2	25	M/F	154
Trapezius, erector spinae	Power Clean	2	15	M/F	142
	Deadlift	2	25	M/F	144
Quadriceps	Squat	2	25	M/F	108
	Lunge	2	25	M/F	110
Latissimus dorsi	Machine Pull-Down	2	25	M/F	152

CLOSING SET

Any exercise described in this book can increase muscular endurance (anaerobic power). The key to increasing a muscle's endurance is the number and resistance level of repetitions performed, and the rest periods between sets.

Muscular endurance is highly specific. Only the muscles trained for increased muscular endurance will demonstrate a marked improvement in muscular endurance. Having followed identical training programs, the stronger of two athletes will demonstrate greater muscular endurance or anaerobic power in the trained movements.

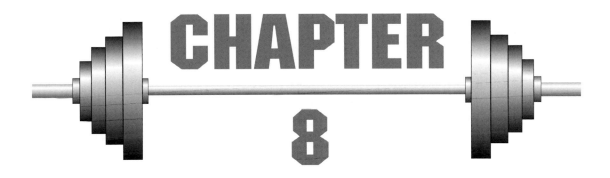

More Muscle Mass

Arnold Schwarzenegger never entered a weight lifting contest. He wasn't strong enough to beat even an average competitive weightlifter. But he sure had lots of muscle—enough to be the best bodybuilder in the world.

Arnold illustrates the point that maximum muscle and maximum strength aren't intractably bound. Yes, bigger muscles *imply* stronger muscles, but there is no definitive correlation between size and strength.

There *is* a definitive correlation between training programs and results. In other words, train one way for maximum muscle, train differently for maximum strength. Although both training protocols produce both larger muscles and more strength, each has an emphasis; maximum muscle or maximum strength.

Bodybuilding seeks maximum muscle at the expense of maximum strength. Strength training seeks maximum strength at the expense of maximum muscle growth. If we throw muscular endurance into the mix, both maximum muscle and strength would be sacrificed in a training program designed to maximize muscular endurance.

If your goal is maximum muscle, you are a bodybuilder—and this is your chapter. Read it, and follow the training program it describes.

WANT BIG ARMS? WORK THE LEGS

Often, a young weight trainer's first question upon entering a gym is, "How can I get bigger arms?" The answer, "Work your legs," sounds like a joke at the novice's expense. It's no joke, though—as the following scenario points out.

◆ Given: Two bodybuilders execute *identical upper body training programs.* One of the bodybuilders does *no leg training.* The other bodybuilder *consistently trains his legs* as part of his overall workout program.

◆ Results: After months of training, the two bodybuilders show *markedly different gains in upper body muscle mass.* The bodybuilder who included leg training in his workout added more upper body muscle to the arms, chest, and shoulders.

How does training the legs correlate to more muscle for the arms, chest, and shoulders? As one possible explanation, scientists point to the temporary elevation of circulating growth hormone brought about by intense leg training. That's right! Intense leg training stimulates a temporary increase in the body's production of growth hormone. This temporary increase in the production of growth hormone is part of the body's natural, adaptive response to training stress.

Now to the connection between the increased production of growth hormone and bigger arms. Once produced by the stimulus of leg training, the growth hormone enters the bloodstream. The elevated blood level of growth hormone reaches every muscle cell of the body—not only the muscles of the legs, but the muscles of the arms, too. The bottom line is that growth hormone is a stimulus to muscle growth. In a simplistic sense, the more growth hormone that reaches a muscle cell, the greater the potential growth.

Referring once again to our two hypothetical bodybuilders, the leg-training bodybuilder grows bigger biceps because the muscle cells of his biceps received more muscle-building growth hormone. You might ask why this extra surge of growth hormone is stimulated by intense leg training, but not by intense biceps training. It's probably because intense leg training (e.g., squats) demands the effort of so much muscle at one time. From head to toe, a heavy squat depends on most of your body's muscle mass. Subjecting all this muscle mass to an intense movement apparently triggers the production of more growth hormone. In contrast, a biceps curl works too little muscle mass to switch on an appreciable production response.

Why don't more wanna-be bodybuilding champions reach their goals? It's a lack of leg training. Whatever the scientific basis, the anecdotal evidence is overwhelming: If you want to be a big-armed champion bodybuilder, spend time on your legs.

THE "PUMP-UP": EXTRA ENERGY FOR WORKING MUSCLES

When a battle breaks out at a corner of a fort, the commander no doubt will send reinforcements racing to the trouble spot. Similarly, your body will send more blood to support the contractions of your biceps when you're curling a dumbbell than when you're leisurely reading this book. That extra blood to the intensely contracting biceps is the bodybuilder's "pump."

Let's take a closer look. Automobiles, light bulbs, and muscles require a constant flow of energy to keep working. Depending on the system, that energy is delivered via streams of gasoline, electricity, or blood. The stream's function is to deliver needed energy. The greater the energy need, the greater the volume of gasoline, electricity, or blood delivered. Unlike the other two energy delivery systems, the bloodstream has the additional responsibility of removing waste products. The science behind the change isn't fully understood, but there is no question that the temporary pump helps build larger muscles.

Your path to a pumped-up biceps is a complicated odyssey of related events. Your heartbeat quickens, increasing the volume of blood into your arteries. Simultaneously, the blood vessels within your muscles open wider to accept the increased flow of blood. What causes this widening? Simply put, your working biceps release potassium, phosphate, and lactic acid. Like a chain reaction, the release of these chemicals relaxes the lining of the blood vessels supplying the biceps, and the vessels open wider.

About five teaspoons of blood per minute enter each pound of your resting biceps muscle. But when your biceps muscle works hard—as it certainly does during an intense set of curls—as much as *75* teaspoons per pound enters the muscle through the widened vessels. This extra blood means extra pump.

Where does the body find this extra blood for the pumped biceps? As more blood is marshaled to the bulging biceps, the vessels in your nonexercising muscles and internal organs constrict (reduce in diameter), forcing blood out. In fact, your liver and intestines lose as much as 80 percent of their normal blood flow while you're vigorously working your skeletal muscles. You needn't worry, though, because the liver and intestines at rest need only 10 to 20 percent of their normal blood-energy supply. Your body's rerouting of blood flow to working muscles is yet another example of the complex internal interactions that support your muscles' energy demands.

BODYBUILDING: ISOLATION EXERCISES

There's not a single exercise in this book that can't be used to build more muscle mass. In fact, most will be incorporated into your bodybuilding program at one time or another. However, compared to other weight training pursuits, bodybuilding relies more heavily on *isolation exercises,* so-named because they "isolate" a specific movement or muscle group. From another perspective, they could have easily been named *spot training exercises* because they focus on a specific spot, or body part. For example, a biceps curl is an isolation exercise that focuses on the bending of the elbow to exercise the biceps. What happens (or doesn't) to other muscle groups during the curl is of no concern to the exerciser.

Isolation exercises are typically single-joint exercises (the movement is confined to one joint) that work relatively little muscle. As such, they're analogous to a sculptor's fine chisels, the last used in refinement of the work of art.

PROFILE: DAVID HUGHES

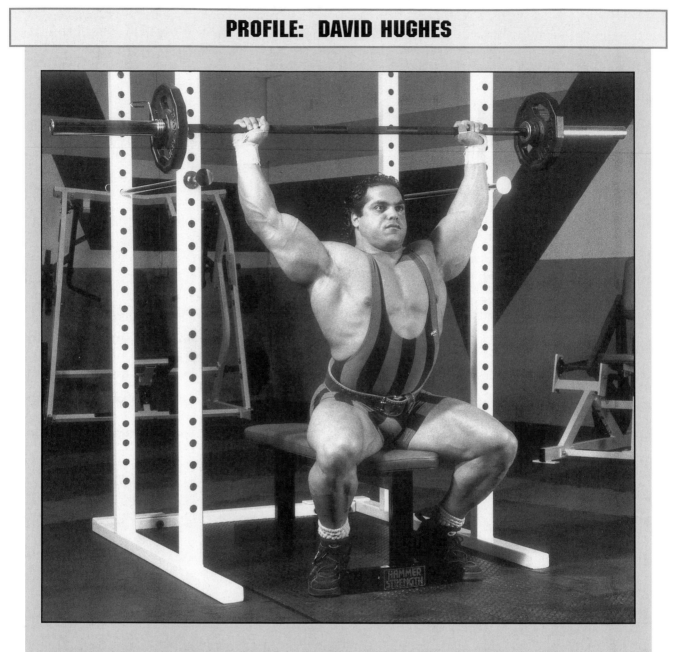

Featured model in *Ironman Magazine*, *Muscular Development*, and *Muscle Magazine*.
Winner of Night of Champions, Redondo Beach, 1994.
Measurements: Arms 22", chest 54", competition weight, 240 lb.
First started bodybuilding in 1989 for Mr. Western Oregon Bodybuilding Championship.

In 1994, Dave won the prestigious 1994 Night of Champions in Redondo Beach, California. "My goal became clear after my first bodybuilding show. I wanted to compete with the best and be able to compete with the best outside of Oregon." The Night of Champions victory took care of that goal.

Dave began lifting weights in high school as an adjunct to football. Like many high school athletes, Dave did lots of work on his chest and arms, but little on his legs. It wasn't until after high school that he began seriously training his legs, and found that serious leg training stimulated enormous upper body growth.

What's Dave's view of training? He enjoys the overall workout, although he used to dislike working his legs. In fact, during the past year, he's gained over two inches on his thighs. One more point: Although he occasionally uses a tape, he feels the best gauge of his overall progress is the mirror.

Competition Diet Schedule

◆ *Starting weight:* 285 lb., goal 240 lbs.

◆ *16 weeks before competition:* "Limit fats; keep calories high, about 5000 calories/day, and portions big." He doesn't drink milk except with morning cereal. His favorite carbohydrate is plain white rice.

◆ *10 weeks before competition:* Cuts out carbohydrates from the last meal. [He doesn't get too stressed out because he allows himself one splurge meal per week during his diet, up until 6 weeks to go.]

◆ *6 weeks to go:* Cut out chicken and turkey and go to fish and egg whites for protein.

Supplements

Takes 1 multivitamin 2-3 times a day; 2,000 mg vitamin C; protein powder drink made with water.

Weekly Routine

4 days on, 1 day off

Day 1: Legs

Day 2: Chest and triceps

Day 3: Back and biceps

Day 4: Shoulders and hamstrings

Sets & Reps

Average 1-2 sets for warm-ups; 3 heavy sets per exercise
8-10 reps upper body; 15 reps for legs
15-20 reps for calves

Exercises

Four exercises for big body parts
Three exercises for smaller parts: biceps and triceps
Abdominals: High Roman chair or rope crunches, 15-20 reps

The converse of isolation exercises are multiple-joint exercises, which involve moving more than one joint at a time. The squat, deadlift, and power clean are typical of the multijoint exercises. They are used to build lots of muscle mass, but in less specific detail. They can't cap the shoulder, sculpt the chest, or peak the biceps—that's the job of isolation exercises.

As noted above, both the traditional, strength-building, multijoint exercises and the sculpting isolation exercises are part and parcel of a bodybuilding program. The multijoint exercises serve as a foundation for a muscular physique, which in turn is to be finely tooled with the isolation exercises.

MUSCLE MASS TRAINING PROGRAMS

A bodybuilding program is neither complicated nor magical: All the basics of sets, reps, exercises, and rest periods are listed in table 8.1. For comparisons to other training programs, turn back to "Weight Training Program Comparisons" on page 62.

TABLE 8.1   The Generic Muscle Mass Building Model

Exercises	Muscle Group	Sets	Reps per Set	Days/ Week
Basic Program	Choose 3	3	8-12	2
Advanced Program	Choose 5	5	8-12	3

Note. These recommendations do not include warm-up sets.

Table 8.1 represents a time-tested exercise protocol that will build a balanced physique—more muscle for all muscle groups. What more should you know?

1. Change the program every six weeks.
2. Change set and rep patterns.

How do you change the program? Merely add and delete exercises for each muscle group. What exercises? That's a personal choice. The important point is to maintain balance. In other words, substitute a leg exercise for another leg exercise. Don't delete a leg exercise and add a biceps exercise.

Set and rep patterns can be changed anytime, as frequently as you want. In fact, *what you want* appears to be the most important factor in determining set-rep patterns. Pick a pattern that is psychologically right for you. One day it might be fewer sets, more reps, and lighter weights. Another day it might be more sets and fewer reps with a heavier weight. Anything within the listed set and rep range is okay.

The most important point of a program change is to select the exercises and set-rep pattern that enhance the prospect of a positive mental approach to the training session, while seeking muscle group balance. The better you feel about training, the harder you'll train and the more dramatic the results you'll achieve.

For your convenience, the exercises in table 8.2, grouped by body part/ muscle group, are done with free weights. Choose three to five exercises per group for your muscle mass workout program. You'll notice that the exercises are labeled "Primary" and "Substitute"; emphasize the primary exercises, but use the substitutes as alternatives to break boredom.

The series of training programs that follow, grouped by body part/muscle group, are done with a combination of free weights and machine exercises. Note also that they do not include warm-ups, so be sure to warm up properly on your own.

TABLE 8.2   Muscle Mass Program Free Weight Exercise Focus

	Primary Exercise		Substitute Exercise	
Legs	◆ Squat	p. 108	◆ Leg Press (if machine available)	p. 106
	◆ Lunge	p. 110	◆ Step-Ups (weighted)	p. 112
	◆ Barbell Seated Calf Raise	p. 120		
Chest	◆ Barbell Bench Press	p. 126	◆ Incline Bench Press	p. 126
	◆ Dumbbell Bench Fly	p. 138	◆ Decline Bench Press	p. 126
	◆ Dip	p. 134		
Back	◆ Deadlift	p. 144	◆ Pull-Ups	p. 150
	◆ Bent-Over Dumbbell Row	p. 156	◆ Bent-Over Barbell Row	p. 158
	◆ Power Clean	p. 142	◆ Seated Long Pull (if machine available)	p. 160
Shoulders	◆ Seated Alternating Overhead Dumbbell Press	p. 166	◆ Barbell Push Press	p. 162
	◆ Alternating Upright Row	p. 170	◆ Upright Row (barbell)	p. 172
	◆ Standing Side Lateral Raises	p. 174	◆ Standing Front Lateral Raises	p. 178
Arms (biceps)	◆ Concentration Biceps Curl	p. 182		
	◆ Barbell Biceps Curl	p. 180		
Arms (triceps)	◆ Lying Barbell Triceps Extension	p. 186	◆ Seated Dumbbell Triceps Extension	p. 188
	◆ Triceps Kickback	p. 192	◆ Barbell Bench Press	p. 126
Abdomen	◆ Sit-Ups	p. 194	◆ Knee-Ups	p. 198

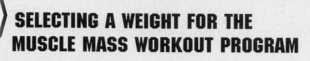

SELECTING A WEIGHT FOR THE MUSCLE MASS WORKOUT PROGRAM

The rule of thumb: Selecting a weight is a matter of trial and error over several workouts because we all have different muscular endurance levels. For each exercise, every individual requires a different weight for his or her 25 repetitions.

If you're a beginner, select your proper weight for each exercise as follows:

◆ With all leg and back exercises, start the experimentation with 10% of your body weight when using both arms and legs.

◆ When using one arm or leg in a lift, even though it seems extremely light, begin the experimentation with 20% of your body weight.

◆ Begin with no added resistance (no weight) when starting the abdominal exercises.

This approach will help you decide if the weight you've selected is too heavy or too light, and you can adjust accordingly over your next several workouts. In several weeks of workouts, you will find what your correct load is for each lift. Caveat—It's better to select too light a weight than too heavy when experimenting to find your correct load.

BIG ARMS PROGRAM

Muscle group	Exercise	Sets	Reps	Days/ week	Page no.
Triceps	Free weight: Lying Barbell Triceps Extension	3-5	8-12	2 per week	186
	Machine: Triceps Extension	3-5	8-12	2 per week	190
Triceps	Free weight: Seated Dumbbell Triceps Extension	3-5	8-12	2 per week	188
Biceps	Free weight: Barbell Biceps Curl	3-5	8-12	2 per week	180
	Machine: Biceps Curl	3-5	8-12	2 per week	184
Biceps	Free weight: Concentration Biceps Curl	3-5	8-12	2 per week	182

WIDER SHOULDERS PROGRAM

Muscle group	Exercise	Sets	Reps	Days/ week	Page no.

Deltoids	Free weight:
	Seated Alternating
	  Overhead Dumbbell
	  Press
		3-5	8-12	2 per week	166

	Machine: Machine Overhead Press	3-5	8-12	2 per week	168
Deltoids	Free weight: Alternating Upright Row	3-5	8-12	2 per week	170
	Machine: Upright Row	3-5	8-12	2 per week	172
Deltoids	Free weight: Standing Front Lateral Raises	3-5	8-12	2 per week	178
Deltoids	Free weight: Dumbbell Shoulder Shrug	3-5	8-12	2 per week	146
	Machine: Shoulder Shrug	3-5	8-12	2 per week	148

BROADER BACK PROGRAM

Muscle group	Exercise	Sets	Reps	Days/ week	Page no.
Latissimus dorsi	Free weight: Bent-Over Dumbbell Row	3-5	8-12	2 per week	156
	Machine: Seated Long Pull	3-5	8-12	2 per week	160
Erector spinae, lower back	Free weight: Deadlift	3-5	8-12	2 per week	144
Latissimus dorsi	Free weight: Pull-Ups	3-5	8-12	2 per week	150
	Machine: Machine Pull-Down	3-5	8-12	2 per week	152
Back	Free weight: Power Clean	3-5	8-12	2 per week	142

MASSIVE CHEST PROGRAM

Muscle group	Exercise	Sets	Reps	Days/week	Page no.
Pectorals	Free weight: Dumbbell Bench Fly	3-5	8-12	2 per week	138
	Machine: Machine Chest Fly	3-5	8-12	2 per week	140
Pectorals	Free weight: Barbell Bench Press	3-5	8-12	2 per week	126
	Machine: Bench Press (Seated or Flat-Back)	3-5	8-12	2 per week	128, 132
Pectorals	Free weight: Incline Barbell Bench Press or Decline Barbell Bench Press	3-5	8-12	2 per week	126
	Machine: Incline Bench Press or Decline Bench Press	3-5	8-12	2 per week	130
Pectorals	Free weight: Dip	3-5	8-12	2 per week	134
	Machine: Dip	3-5	8-12	2 per week	136

ABDOMINALS PROGRAM

Muscle group	Exercise	Sets	Reps	Days/week	Page no.
Abdominals	Free weight: Sit-Ups	3-5	8-12	2 per week	194
Abdominals	Free weight: Knee-Ups	3-5	8-12	2 per week	198
Abdominals	Free weight: Reverse Trunk Twist	3-5	8-12	2 per week	196

THIGHS PROGRAM

Muscle group	Exercise	Sets	Reps	Days/ week	Page no.
Quadriceps	Free weight: Squat	3-5	8-12	2 per week	108
Quadriceps	Free weight: Step-Ups	3-5	8-12	2 per week	112
	Machine: Leg Press	3-5	8-12	2 per week	106
Hamstrings	Machine: Leg Curl (Horizontal or Seated)	3-5	8-12	2 per week	114, 116
Quadriceps	Machine: Leg Extension	3-5	8-12	2 per week	118
Quadriceps, hamstrings	Free weight: Lunge (Barbell or Dumbbell)	3-5	8-12	2 per week	110

CALVES PROGRAM

Muscle group	Exercise	Sets	Reps	Days/ week	Page no.
Calves	Free weight: Barbell Seated Calf Raise	3-5	8-12	2 per week	120
Calves	Machine: Horizontal Calf Raise	3-5	8-12	2 per week	122
Calves	Machine: Calf Raise	3-5	8-12	2 per week	122, 124

CLOSING SET

Any weight training exercise will increase the mass of the muscle being exercised, providing the weight trainer follows an appropriate program of sets, reps, and resistance levels. The programs in this chapter are representative of programs used by bodybuilders to increase the mass and shape of body parts.

All levels of bodysculpters, from twice-weekly circuit trainers to professional bodybuilders, rely on isolation exercises to fine-tune a physique. Overall mass building is more readily accomplished with multijoint exercises because, rep per rep, multijoint exercises work more muscle.

Leg training is an often overlooked program variable. Upper body mass is more easily developed when leg training is an integral part of the weight trainer's program. The "pump" is a natural response to the body's sending more blood, oxygen, and energy to the working muscle.

Just as any exercise can be used to build more muscle mass, any person wanting more muscle can have it through the appropriate application of those exercises. Arnold did it, Dave Hughes did it, and you can do it, too.

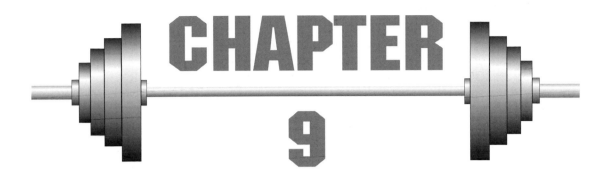

CHAPTER 9

Lifting Techniques and Tips

Each and every exercise in this chapter can be used to change the strength, endurance, and size of the exercised muscle. In short, you have lots of opportunities for exercise variety and specificity to your workouts. First, though, let's review some important considerations pertaining to all exercises.

Is a warm-up important? Yes. For each exercise, a warm-up consisting of one or two sets with a lighter weight (40% of your lightest work set weight) increases blood volume and pliability of the muscles that will be overloaded during the work sets. For example, a warm-up of one or two sets of bench presses with 80 pounds would be employed by a lifter whose first work set is 200 pounds. Throughout the workout, exercise after exercise, the warm-up sets precede the work sets.

Is breath control important? Generally, it's best to train with a natural (i.e., not intentionally altered) breathing cadence. In other words, there is generally no mandated time to "breathe in" or "breathe out." Nor should you hold your breath while lifting. Where breath control is important, it is noted in the exercise description.

Are spotters necessary? For safety, some exercises require a spotter or an apparatus—such as a stop on a machine—that takes the place of a spotter. Such cases will be pointed out in the exercise descriptions.

Machines or free weights? If you have access to both types of equipment, use both for a greater variety of stimuli, perhaps free weights one workout and machines the next. The prime consideration in equipment selection is that the equipment allows the muscle to work through a full and natural range of motion. That's never a problem with free weights, and the machines pictured in this book, manufactured by Hammer Strength, closely duplicate natural movements while allowing a full range of motion. Hammer Strength is the author's choice among available exercise machines. For more information, contact Hammer Strength at P.O. Box 19040, Cincinnati, OH, 45219 (phone 800-543-1123 or 513-221-2600; fax 513-221-8084). For more information about free weights, contact Iron Grip Barbell Company at 10534 Bechler River Avenue, Fountain Valley, CA, 92708 (phone 800-664-4766; fax 714-378-4113).

What about specificity of movement? Specificity of movement comes into play in exercise selection when your motive for weight training is to improve sports performance. In brief, the concept of "specificity" requires that you choose a weight training exercise that most closely mimics the sports movement you're hoping to improve.

For example, the squat (see pages 108-109) generally duplicates the motion of a jump. Hence, the squat brings the specific body mechanics that the athlete might use during the jump into the developmental effort put forth in the weight room. Hence, squats are at the base of a jumper's weight training program.

If your primary goal is not sports performance, don't concern yourself with the concept of specificity. If improved sports performance *is* your reason for weight training, choose the weight training exercises that most closely mimic the sporting movements you're trying to improve.

Multijoint or isolation exercises? Multijoint exercises, such as a power clean (see pages 142-143), involve the muscles responsible for the movement of more than one joint. On the other hand, isolation exercises, such as the leg extension (see pages 118-119), work through a single joint. As you might suspect, multijoint exercises work more muscle per repetition.

The appropriateness of multijoint or isolation exercises depends on numerous factors, but there are several general guidelines. Isolation exercises are best at building (or remediating) the strength, endurance, or size of a specific muscle group: They allow the weight trainer to narrowly focus her attention and effort.

Multijoint exercises are usually at the foundation of training programs designed for increasing overall strength, endurance, or size. In fact, a complete, full-body workout can be accomplished with a handful of multijoint exercises.

Chances are that both multijoint and isolation exercises will, at one time or another, be regular features of your workout program.

How are exercises grouped in this chapter? The exercises are grouped by body part or muscle group.

Multijoint exercises—those involving more than one body part or muscle group—are listed according to the muscle group traditionally emphasized during the exercise movement. For example, the power clean, although involving numerous muscle groups and body parts, is listed with back exercises since weight trainers have traditionally used power cleans primarily to work the back.

How are "Muscles Emphasized" prioritized? The muscles listed under "Muscles Emphasized" are prioritized according to the importance of the given exercise on training a specific muscle group.

For example, the squat involves most of the body's muscle mass, but when prioritizing the intended training benefit of the squat, the order goes like this: quadriceps, gluteals, erector spinae, hamstrings, and abdominals. Of course, the squat incorporates the trapezius, soleus, and so on, but those are the inconsequential benefits of the exercise—hence, not listed under "Muscles Emphasized."

Keep these considerations in mind as you review and perform the exercises on pages 106-199.

Leg Press

Muscles Emphasized: Quadriceps, gluteals, and hamstrings.

Exercise Technique

1. Sit on the machine seat and put your feet on the platform. Position your back against the back rest. Your feet must be perfectly flat on the foot platform, spaced 18 to 24 inches apart. The seat should be adjusted so that your thighs are as close as possible to your chest.

2. Grasp the handles on the seat to help stabilize your body.

3. Press forward with your legs until the legs are fully extended. Do not hyperextend the legs.

4. Slowly and smoothly lower weight to the bottom position. Avoid bouncing the weight down.

5. Keep the hips down and the lower back pressed against the back rest during the entire movement.

6. Press the weight to the top position.

Note. *The leg press requires a machine. The closest free weight equivalent exercise is the squat.*

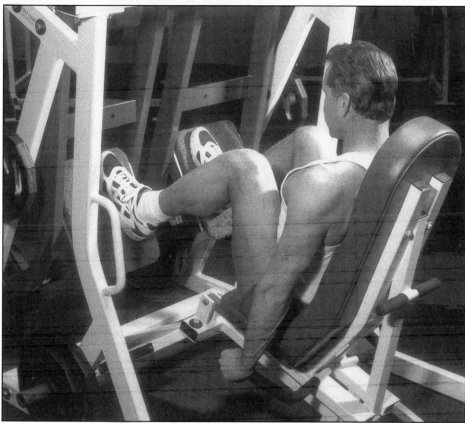

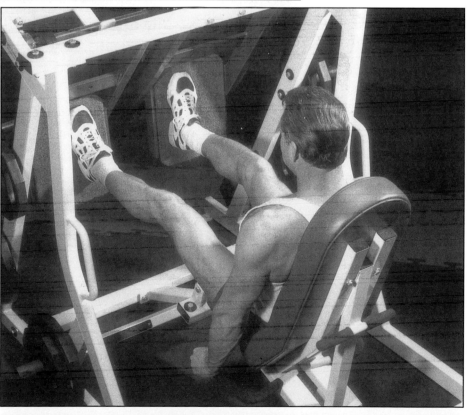

Squat

Muscles Emphasized: Quadriceps, gluteals, hamstrings, erector spinae, and abdominals.

Exercise Technique

1. Stand with your feet shoulder width apart, bar held in a resting position across the shoulders. Isometrically contracting the abdominals and back muscles (i.e., tensing the muscles) will help stabilize your torso.

2. Keeping the heels in contact with floor and eyes forward, lower to the bottom position without bending the trunk forward more than necessary (less than 45 degrees).

3. Without stopping at the bottom position, drive up to the starting position. Do not bounce or jerk at the bottom position. Although there is technically a stop at the juncture of down and up, the reversal of directions is a smooth transition.

Training Tip

Squat until your thighs are parallel to the floor. It's important that your heels remain on the floor during the entire movement, keeping your knees above your feet. Lifting the heels propels the knees forward, subjecting the knee to undesirable forces.

Spotter Needed! Have a spotter standing by to assist the completion of the lift, especially if you're squatting outside the safety bars of a power rack.

Breath Control Alert! Don't inflate your lungs and hold your breath during this movement: The inflated lungs, and the torso's flexed muscles (and maybe a belt), constrict blood flow, possibly raising blood pressure to extreme levels.

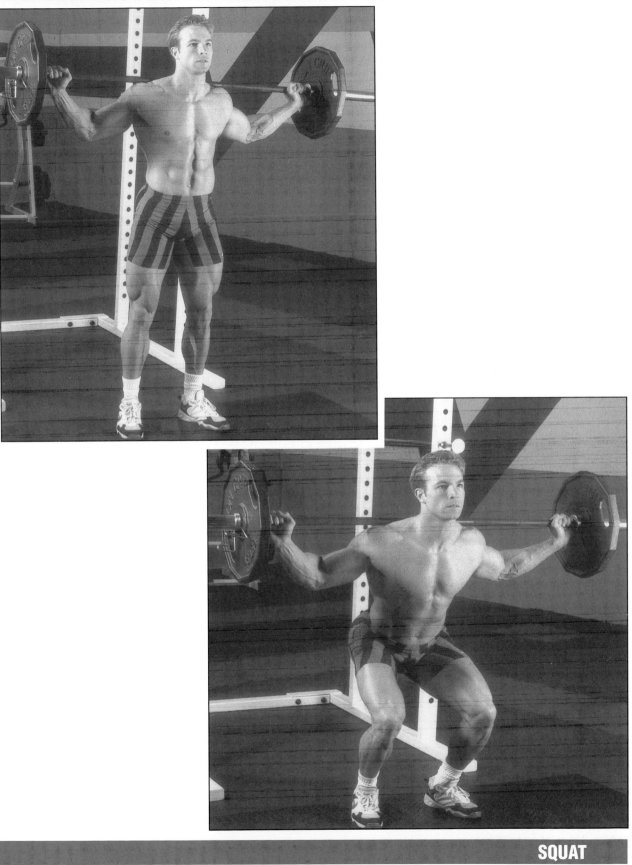

SQUAT

Lunge

Muscles Emphasized: Quadriceps of the frontal thighs, gluteals of the buttocks, and hamstrings; lesser emphasis on erector spinae, calves, and abdominals.

Exercise Technique

1. Stand upright with feet placed shoulder width apart. Hold dumbbells at arm's length, palms facing toward thighs, or firmly grip a barbell positioned on your shoulders.

2. Keeping head up and back straight, take a long step forward with either foot. Plant the foot and drop the hips until the lead thigh is parallel to the floor.

3. Push backward and upward with the lead foot until you are standing erect at the starting position.

4. Repeat with the opposite leg. That's one rep.

Training Tip

Keep your front heel on the ground as you drop into the low position; doing so helps keep your front knee above your foot, protecting the knee.

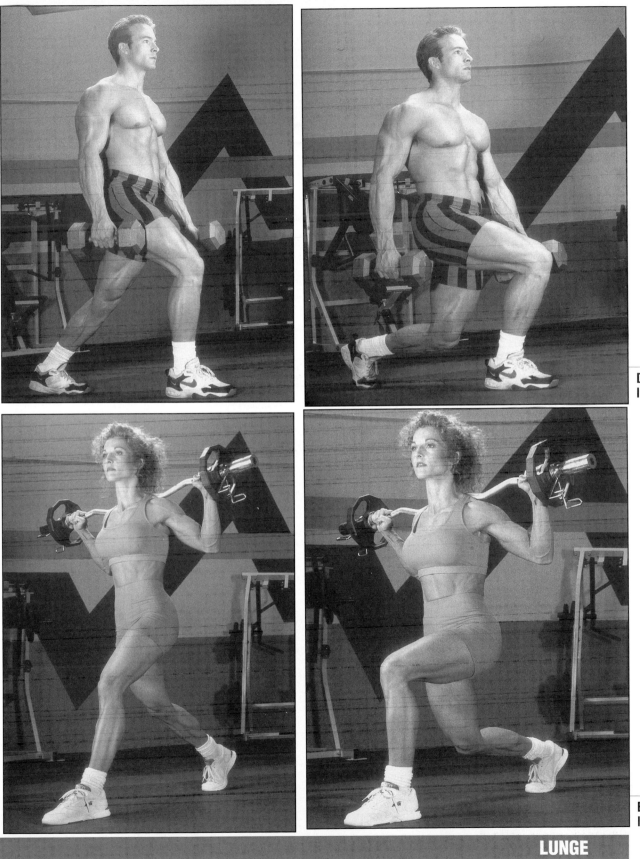

Dumbbell lunge.

Barbell lunge.

LUNGE

Step-Ups

Muscles Emphasized: Quadriceps at the fronts of the thighs, the gluteal muscles of the buttocks, hip flexors, hamstrings, lower back, calves, and abdominals.

Exercise Technique

1. With feet together, stand facing the end of the weight bench, holding a barbell across your shoulders.
2. Step up with the left foot, standing erect on top of the bench.
3. Step down to the floor, starting with the right leg and trailing with the left.
4. Repeat the movement, stepping up with the right leg and continuing the sequence. That's a rep.
5. Continue to alternate legs until you've completed the required number of reps. That's a set.

Safety Tip

Check your bench for stability before beginning this exercise.

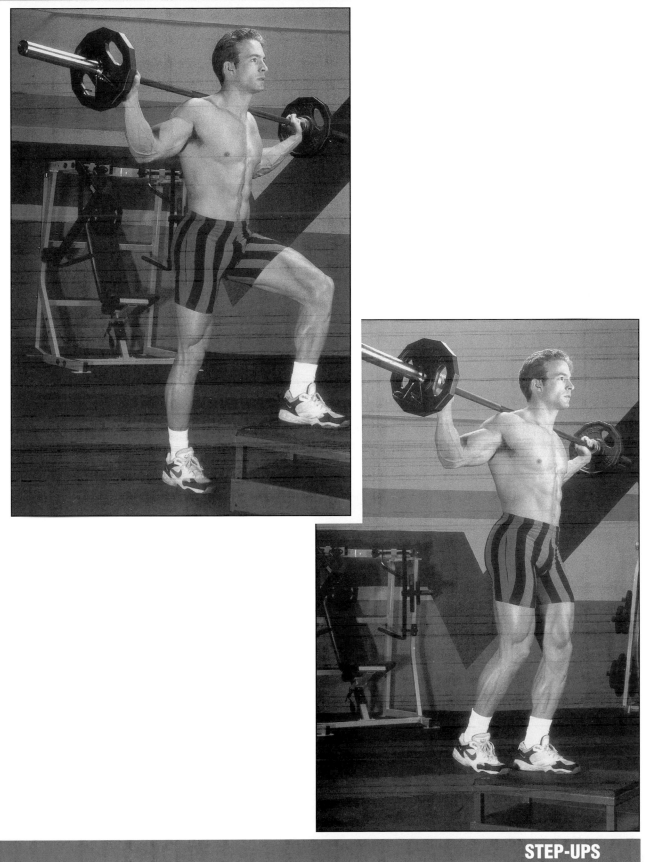

Horizontal Machine Leg Curl

Muscles Emphasized: Hamstrings at rear of thigh.

Exercise Technique

1. Lie face down on the machine, positioning the leg pad at the back of the ankles.
2. Without jerking or raising your hips from the bench, bend one or both legs at the knee while concentrating on the contraction of your hamstrings.
3. Under control, lower to the starting position.

Training Tip

Keep your hips pressed against the bench to ensure that the leg biceps travel a full range of motion. Perform the exercise one leg at a time for a little variety.

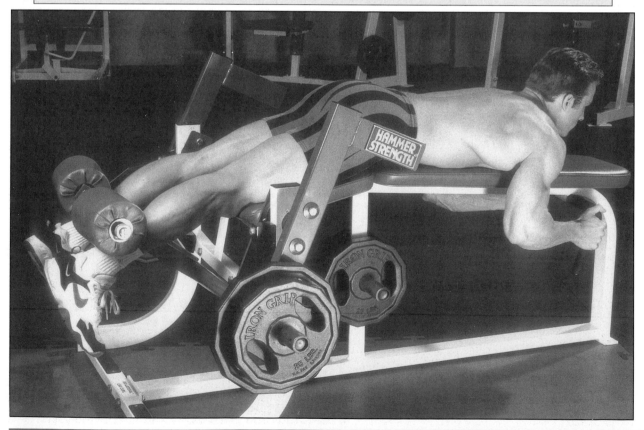

HORIZONTAL MACHINE LEG CURL

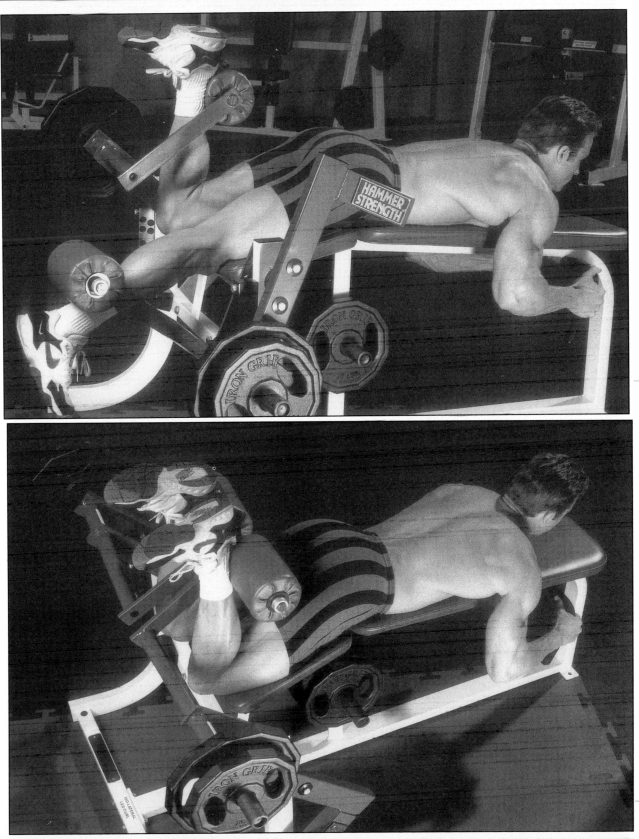

Single-
leg curl.

Double-
leg curl.

HORIZONTAL MACHINE LEG CURL

Seated Machine Leg Curl

An alternative to the horizontal machine leg curl.

Muscles Emphasized: Hamstrings at rear of thigh.

Exercise Technique

1. Sit on seat, grip handles, and press your back against the pad. Position your legs up on the cushion, resting your calves against the pad.
2. Curl legs downward and back.
3. Pause, then raise your legs slowly to starting position.

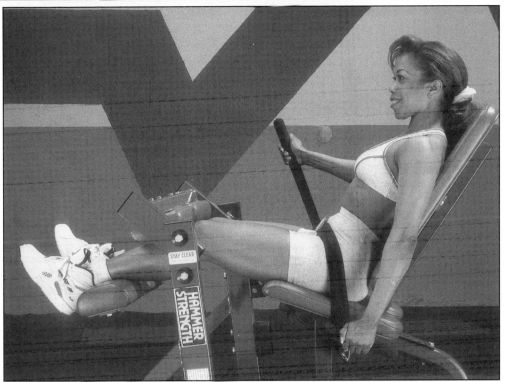

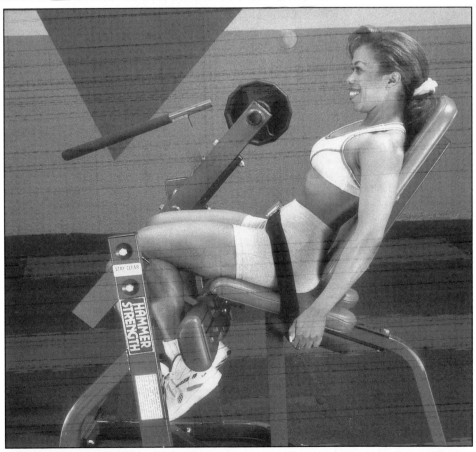

Leg Extension

Muscles Emphasized: Quadriceps at front of thigh.

Exercise Technique

1. Sit in the machine with ankles behind and pressed against the ankle pad.
2. Without jerking to accelerate the weight, straighten your legs until your knees are locked.
3. Lower your legs to the starting position, completely stopping at the bottom. That's a rep.

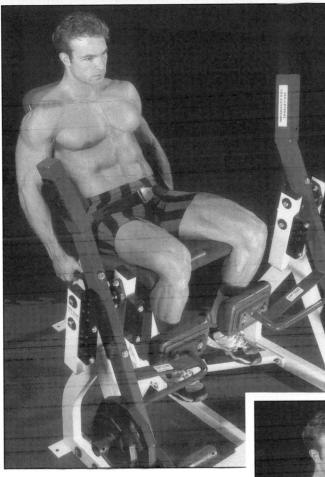

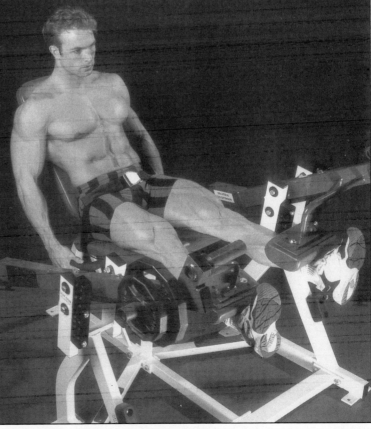

Barbell Seated Calf Raise

Muscles Emphasized: Soleus and gastrocnemius of the calf.

Exercise Technique

1. Sit on the bench with your toes on the footboard and a barbell across the tops of the knees.

2. Raise up your heels with resistance by the barbell.

3. Under control, return to the heels-low position. That's a rep.

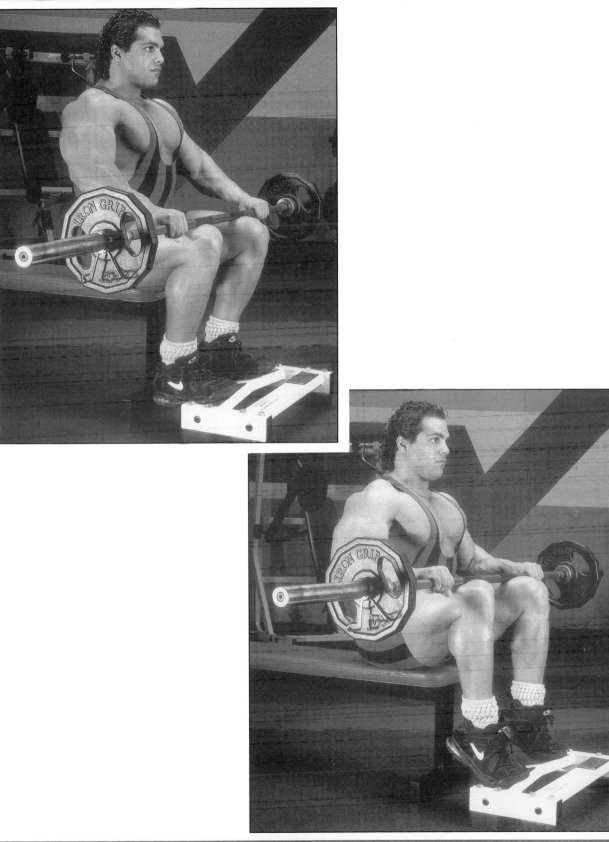

BARBELL SEATED CALF RAISE

Horizontal Calf Raise Machine

An alternative to the barbell seated calf raise.

Muscles Emphasized: Gastrocnemius of the calf.

Exercise Technique

1. Seated in the machine, legs extended, resistance on the balls of the feet, extend the ankle.
2. Under control, maintaining a straight leg, bend the ankle as far as possible.
3. Press to the extended position to repeat the movement.

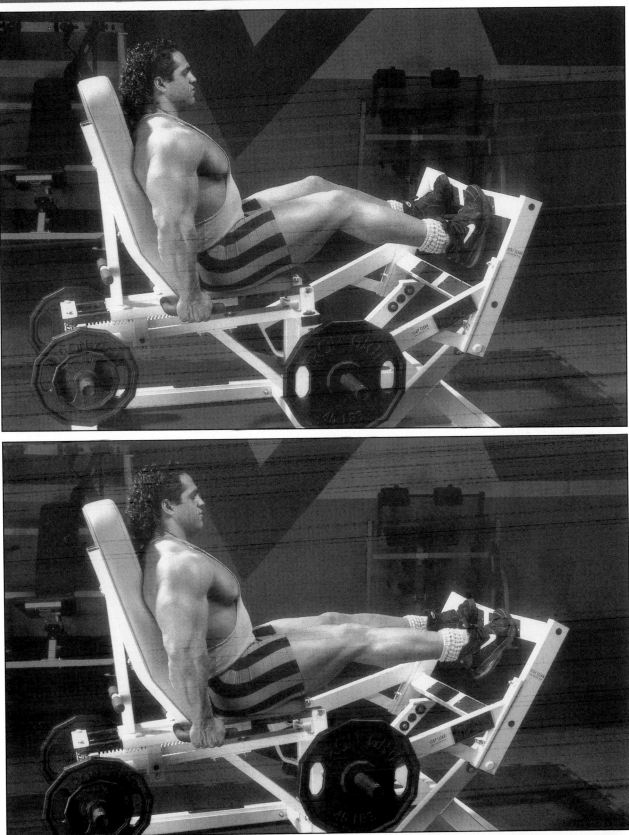

HORIZONTAL CALF RAISE MACHINE

Seated Calf Raise Machine

Muscles Emphasized: Soleus and gastrocnemius of the calf.

Exercise Technique

1. Seated, knee pad in place, the balls of your feet on the footpad, stretch your calves by lowering the heels. That's the starting position.

2. Raise up on the toes as high as possible, momentarily holding the contraction of your calf muscles at the top.

3. Under control, lower your heels to the stretched-calf starting position. That's a rep.

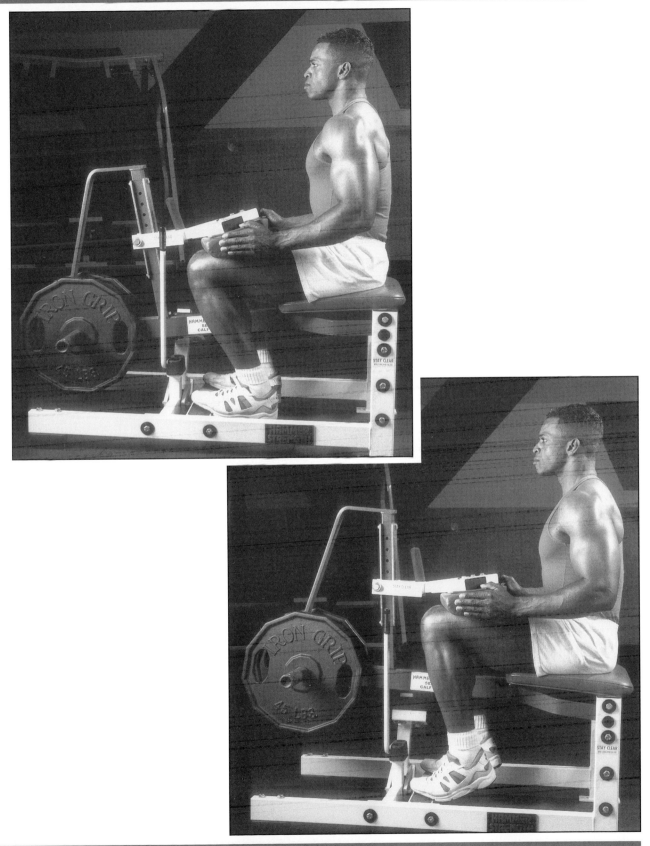

Barbell Bench Press

Muscles Emphasized: Pectorals; lesser emphasis on deltoids and triceps.

Exercise Technique

1. Start with your feet firmly planted on the floor, hands shoulder-width apart, bar supported at arm's length.
2. The bar remains under control as it is lowered to the chest with elbows out. If using a flat bench, the bar should touch the chest an inch above the nipples; high on the chest if using an incline bench; and below the nipples if using a decline bench.
3. Press the bar up until the arms are extended.

Training Tips

Workout to workout, change the bench angles—flat, incline, or decline. Multiple bench angles varies the exercise stimulus, broadening the potential range of muscular adaptation.

As with bench angles, occasionally vary hand spacing from shoulder width to near-collar width to further enhance the potential range of adaptation.

Spotter Alert! The free weight bench press is a must for a spotter: Imagine being exhausted and pinned under a heavy weight!

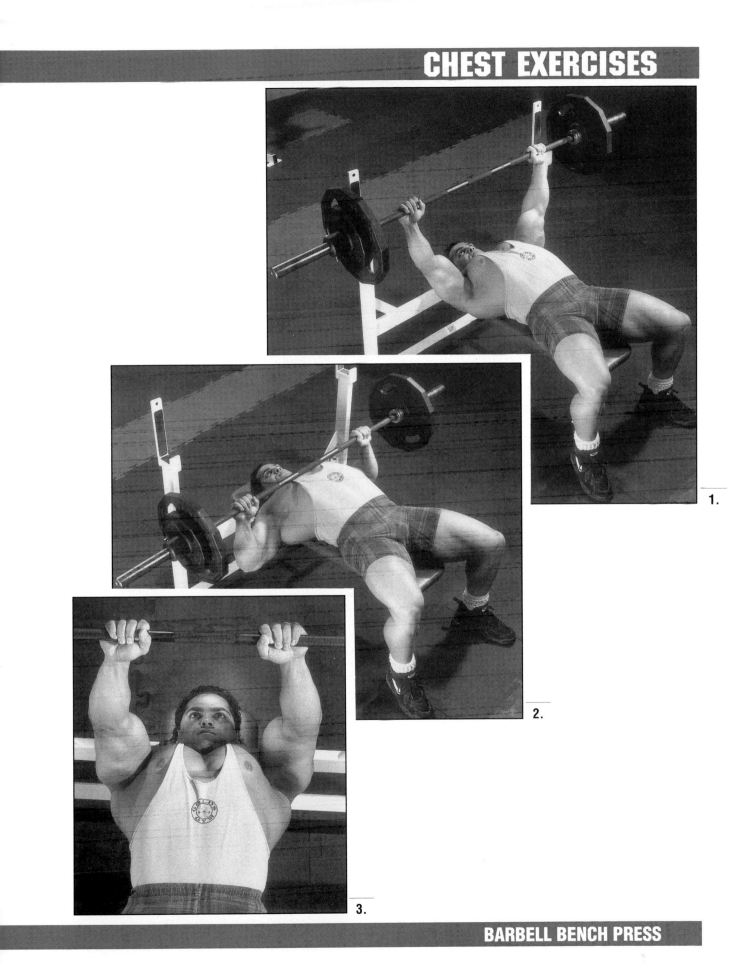

1.

2.

3.

BARBELL BENCH PRESS

Seated Machine Bench Press

An alternative to the barbell bench press.

Muscles Emphasized: Pectorals, deltoids, and triceps. The pictured bench press machine, the Hammer Strength Iso-Lateral Bench Press, allows for double-arm or single-arm movement. Always check the manufacturer's plaque mounted on the machine for the manufacturers' suggested use, as instructions will vary.

Exercise Technique: Exercise technique and results are similar to those of the barbell bench press.

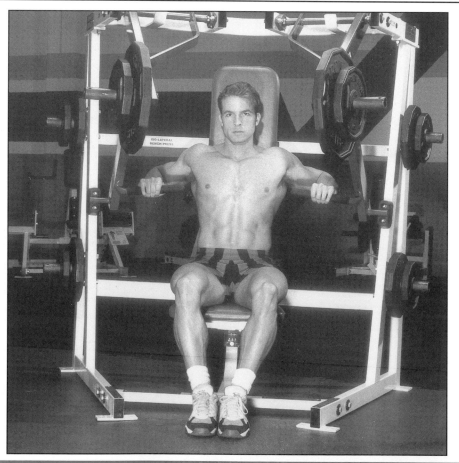

SEATED MACHINE BENCH PRESS

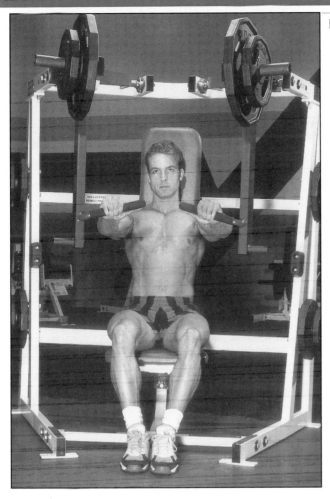

Double-arm press.

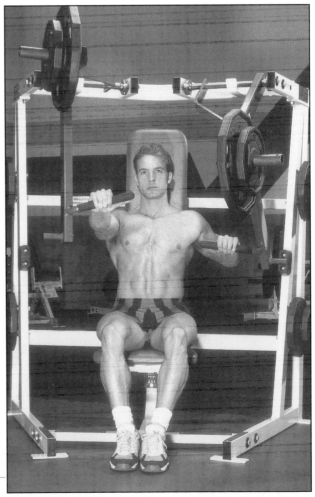

Single-arm press.

SEATED MACHINE BENCH PRESS

Machine Incline Bench Press

An alternative to the bench press.

The pictured machine allows for a movement angle different from that of a typical bench press movement. In the illustrated example, the arms are moving at a 45-degree angle to the chest. The different movement angle adds variety and a different adaptational response by the muscles. Once again, the machine allows for double-arm or single-arm movement.

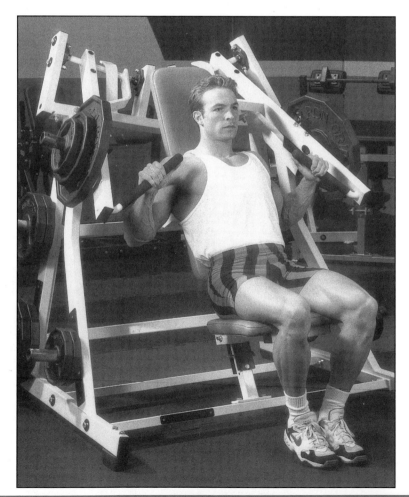

MACHINE INCLINE BENCH PRESS

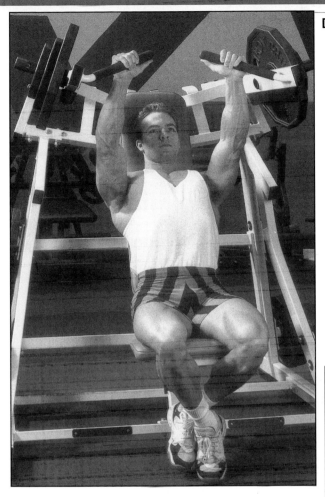

Double-arm press.

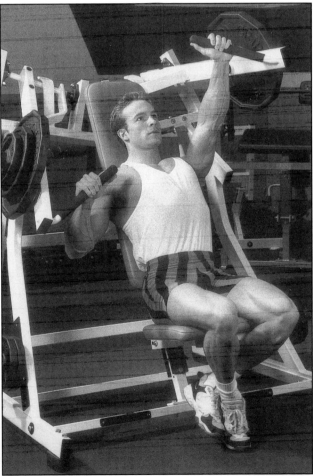

Single-arm press.

Machine Flat-Back Bench Press

An alternative to the bench press.

A flat-back bench press machine is another configuration available from some manufacturers. The pictured machine, analogous to the barbell bench press, has the added advantage of variety, allowing for single-arm movements.

Training Tip

The pictured machine offers the advantages of dumbbells (i.e., single-arm movements) and the safety of a machine. Compared to barbells, or an equivalent two-arm machine, single-arm movements permit a more natural, pressing movement and a greater range of motion during the pressing exercise. For an athlete, the dumbbell bench press is the superior exercise.

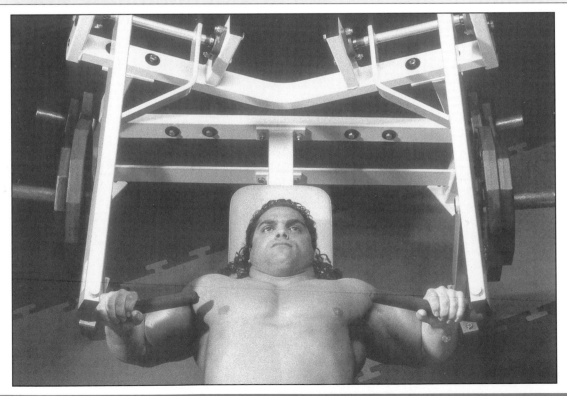

MACHINE FLAT-BACK BENCH PRESS

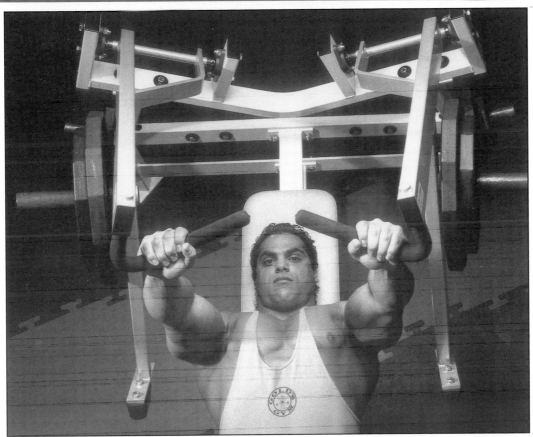

Double-arm press.

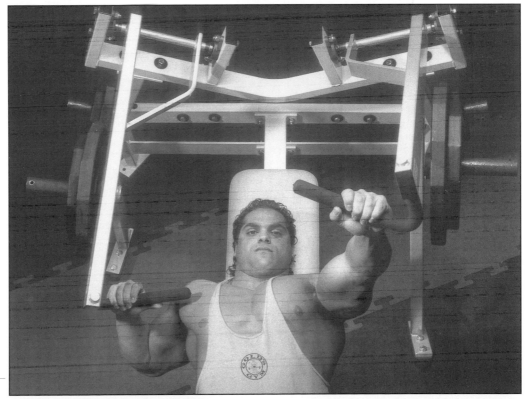

Single-arm press.

MACHINE FLAT-BACK BENCH PRESS

Dip

Muscles Emphasized: Lower pectorals, deltoids, triceps, upper pectorals, and latissimus dorsi.

Exercise Technique

1. Start the exercise by supporting yourself on dip bars, arms straight and shoulder width apart, body in an erect position with eyes forward.

2. Bend your elbows, lowering your body under control until you feel a stretch in your shoulder muscles. Your elbows should point in the direction of the bar. [If the bars are straight, the elbows should point straight back; if the dip bars are angled, the elbows should follow the angle of the bar.]

3. Press upward until you have reached the starting position. That's a rep.

Training Tip

If your equipment is adjustable, vary the angle of the dip bars or widen the placement of your hands on the dip bar from workout to workout.

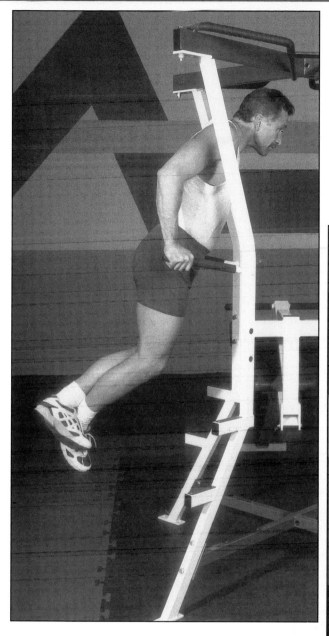

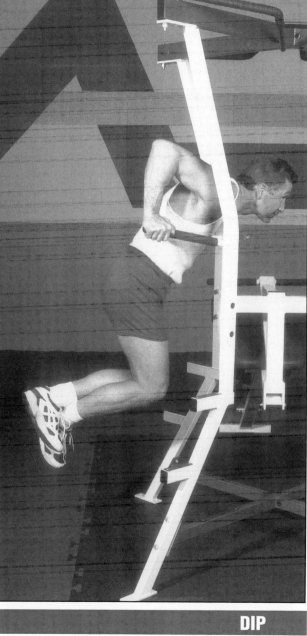

Machine Dip

An alternative to the free bar dip.

Muscles Emphasized: Lower pectorals, deltoids, triceps, upper pectorals, and latissimus dorsi.

Exercise Technique

1. Adjust seat so that arms are parallel to floor when you are seated; sit and attach belt.
2. Press downward, extending the elbows until arms are straight.
3. Under control, return to the starting position. That's a rep.

Note. A machine dip offers the advantage of widely adjustable resistance—resistance both greater and less than your body weight.

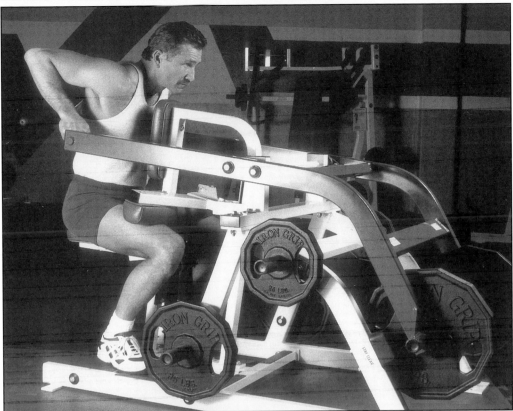

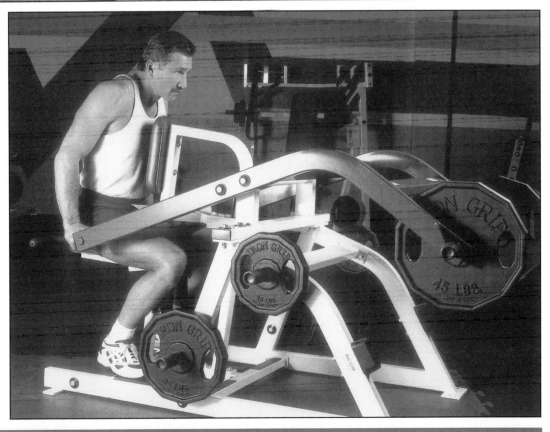

Dumbbell Bench Fly

Muscles Emphasized: Pectorals and deltoids.

Exercise Technique

1. Lie on a flat, incline, or decline bench, with your feet flat on the floor. Hold the dumbbells at arm's length above the shoulders, palms facing each other as the dumbbells nearly touch.

2. Lower the dumbbells through semicircles until the shoulders and chest are comfortably stretched. The elbows can bend as much as 45 degrees while lowering the dumbbells.

3. Return the dumbbells to the starting position through the same semicircular path, being careful not to bang the dumbbells at the top. That's a rep.

Spotter Alert! Until the coordination for the movement has been perfected, beginners should avail themselves of an experienced spotter to guide them through the arc of the exercise movement.

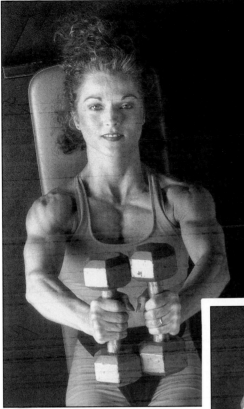

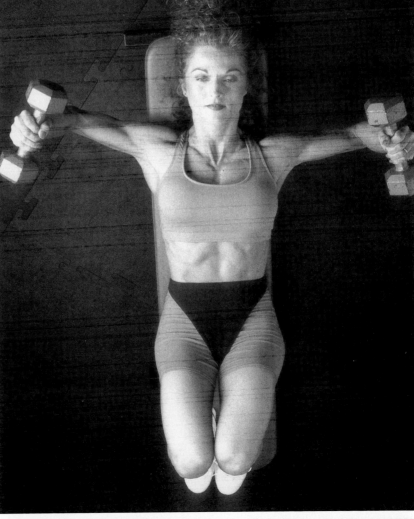

DUMBBELL BENCH FLY

Machine Chest Fly

An alternative to the dumbbell bench fly.

Muscles Emphasized: Pectorals and deltoids.

Exercise Technique

1. Lie on back, head higher than hips, pads in crooks of elbows.
2. Raise your arms in semicircular movements until the pads touch over your chest.
3. Return under control to starting position.

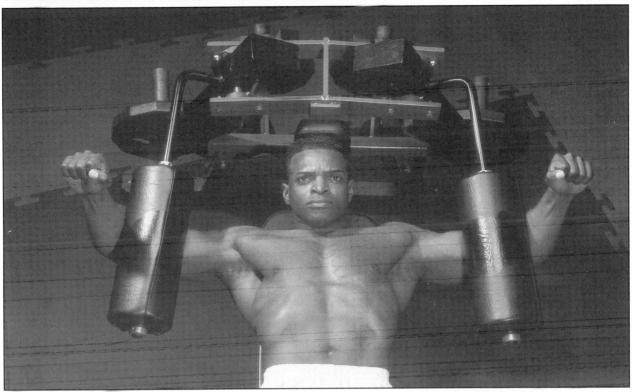

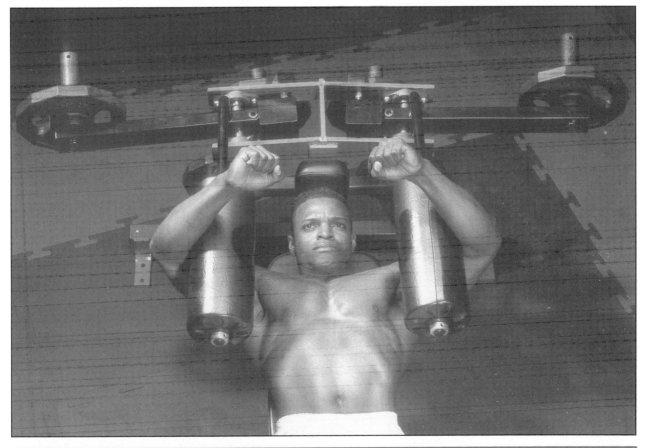

Power Clean

Muscles Emphasized: Trapezius, erector spinae, latissimus dorsi of the back; quadriceps, hamstrings, gluteals, biceps, deltoids, forearms, and calves.

Exercise Technique

1. Stand with feet apart, shins touching the bar. Bend down and take an overhand grip on the bar. Upper legs are parallel to the floor, the back is straight, and the eyes are looking forward.

2. Straightening the legs, keep your arms straight as the barbell is lifted from the floor.

3. As the legs straighten, the hips extend forward, initiating an erect posture. The arms begin to bend at this point.

4. As the body reaches an erect posture, continue the ascent of the bar by simultaneously pulling with the arms and rising on the toes until the bar reaches the highest possible point.

5. When the bar reaches its highest point, bend the knees, catching the bar on the shoulders and upper chest. Straighten to a standing position.

6. Control the bar, lowering it to the floor. That's a rep.

Training Tip

Heavy power cleans require mastering the leg/hip/arm sequence of the pull. Acceleration of the barbell is initiated by powerful leg and lower back muscles. The less powerful muscles of the upper body can complete the movement. Reread "Quick Lifts" in chapter 6 for more information.

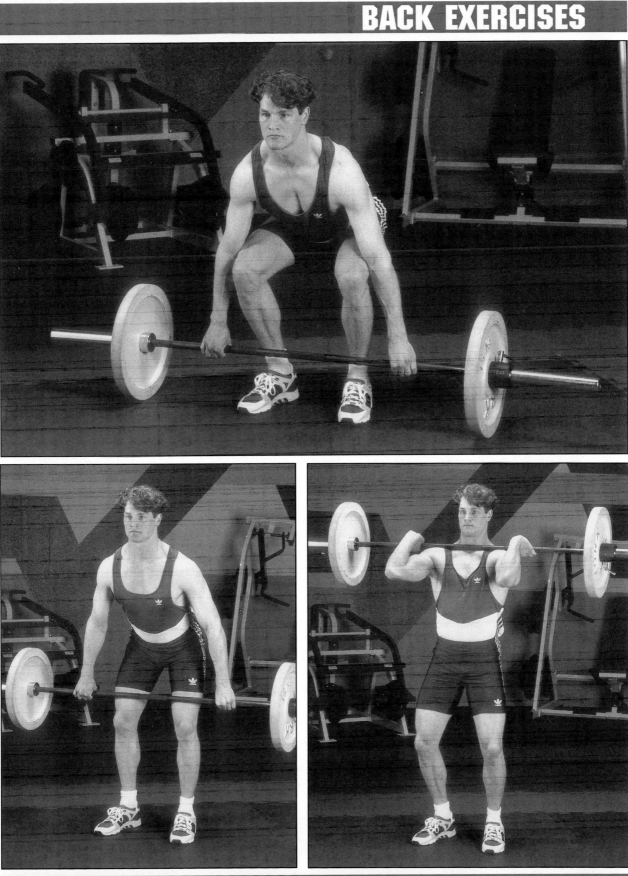

POWER CLEAN

Deadlift

Muscles Emphasized: Erector spinae, trapezius, latissimus dorsi, quadriceps, forearms, hamstrings, hip extensors.

Exercise Technique

1. Start with feet about shoulder-width apart, shins touching the bar, toes slightly pointed outward. Grip the bar at shoulder width. Keeping your back as erect as possible, bend your knees until your thighs are parallel to the floor. Look straight ahead throughout the deadlift.

2. Pull the barbell upward, simultaneously straightening your legs and extending the hips forward until your body is erect. While straightening your legs and extending your hips, keep the bar close to the body. When your body is erect, the barbell should rest against the thighs.

3. Looking straight ahead, lower the barbell by simultaneously bending the hips and the knees as the bar is returned to the floor. Maintain control of the bar throughout the exercise, keeping it as close to the body as possible. That's a rep.

Beginner's Tip

Don't jerk the weight from the floor or bounce the weight on the floor between reps. Form is critical.

Training Tip

Work on your range of motion. Stand atop a low platform to extend the movement several additional inches if your flexibility permits.

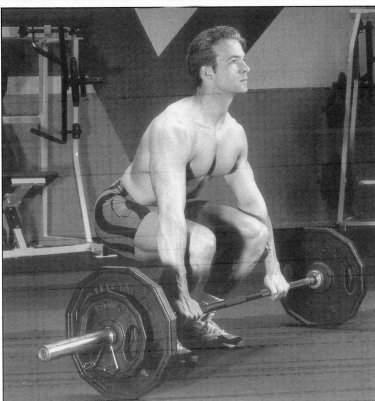

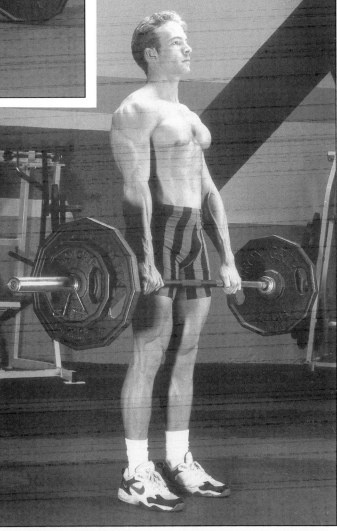

Dumbbell Shoulder Shrug

Muscles Emphasized: Trapezius.

Exercise Technique

1. Stand erect, holding a pair of dumbbells hanging at your sides.
2. Raise the shoulders as high as possible while keeping the arms straight.
3. Lower the shoulders to the starting position. That's a rep.

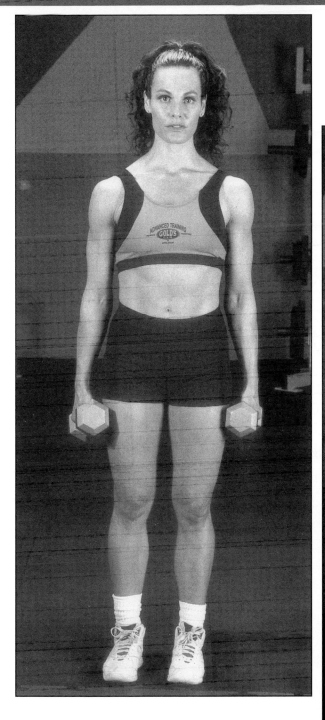

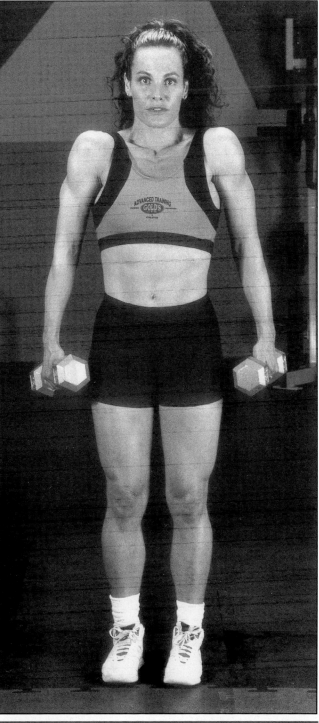

DUMBBELL SHOULDER SHRUG

Machine Shoulder Shrug

An alternative to the dumbbell shoulder shrug.

Muscles Emphasized: Trapezius.

Exercise Technique

1. Stand erect holding the machine handles, arms hanging at your sides.
2. Raise the shoulders as high as possible while keeping the arms straight.
3. Lower the shoulders to the starting position. That's a rep.

Exercise Tip

Don't bend your arms while performing the shrug movement. Bending the elbow lets the biceps do some of the pulling, relieving the trapezius of the full load.

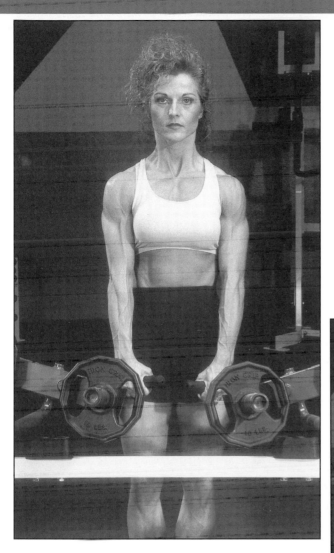

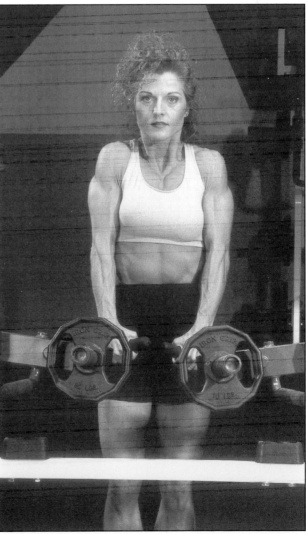

MACHINE SHOULDER SHRUG

Pull-Ups

Muscles Emphasized: Latissimus dorsi, deltoids, biceps, and forearms.

Exercise Technique

1. Start by hanging from the bar with your choice of a hand grip. Hang as low as possible, fully stretching the lats, arms, and shoulders.
2. Pull your body up until eye level with the bar.
3. Lower to the starting position. That's a rep.

Exercise Tip

Resistance can be increased by wearing a weighted belt or decreased by having a training partner assist the movement.

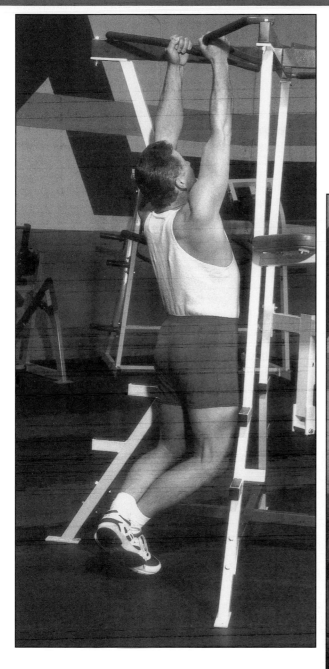

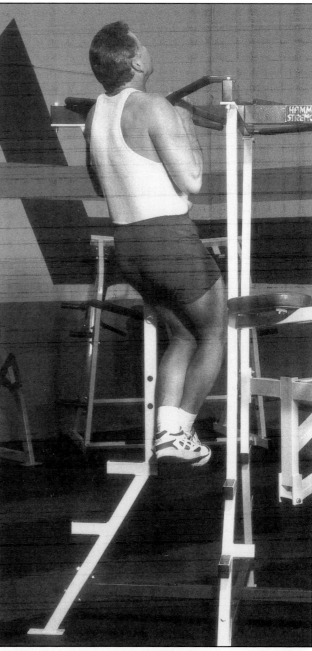

Machine Pull-Down

An alternative to pull-ups.

Muscles Emphasized: Latissimus dorsi, deltoids, biceps, and forearms.

Exercise Technique

1. Sitting with your legs under a bracing bar, pull the handles down until they touch the top of your chest.
2. Under control, return the handles to the starting position. That's a rep.

Training Tip

Workout to workout, vary your hand spacing. The varied hand spacing stimulates a broader range of muscular adaptation. Occasionally add variety with single-arm pull-downs.

Note. *A pull-down machine has a distinct advantage over the free bar pull-up. The pull-down machine allows for greater or less than body weight resistance, while working the same muscle groups.*

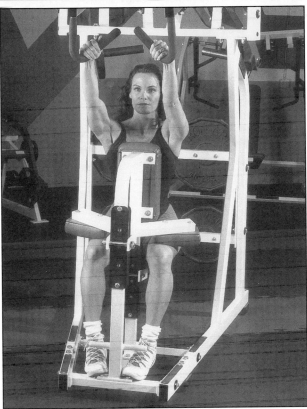

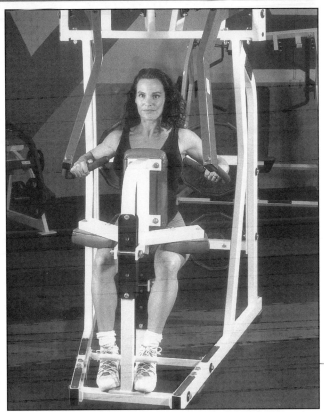

Double-arm pull-down.

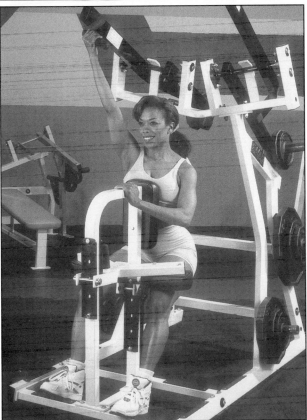

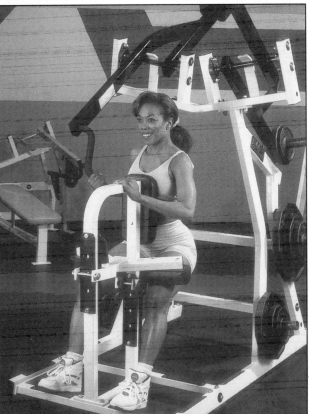

Single-arm pull-down.

MACHINE PULL-DOWN

Back Extension

Muscles Emphasized: Erector spinae, buttocks, and hamstrings.

Exercise Technique

1. Stand erect, barbell firmly positioned on your shoulders, feet shoulder-width apart, and knees slightly bent.

2. Keep your back straight, and bend at the waist until your torso is perpendicular to your legs. Your knees will naturally bend more to maintain your balance.

3. Return to the starting position, maintaining a straight back throughout the arc of movement. Hold the starting position for a second. That's a rep.

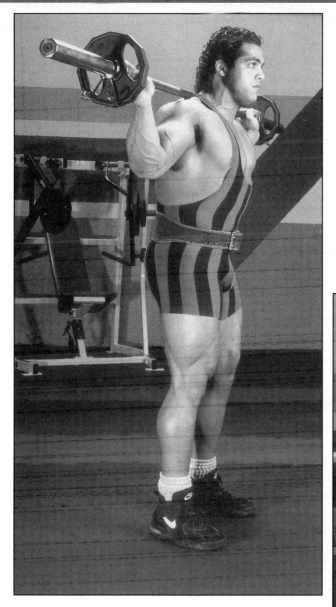

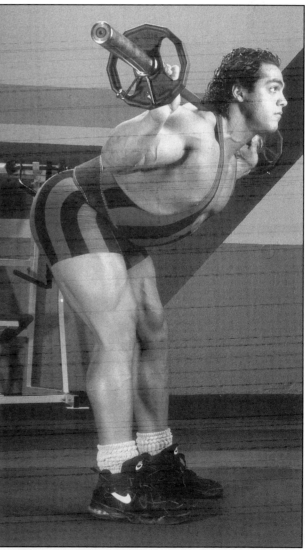

BACK EXTENSION

Bent-Over Dumbbell Row

Muscles Emphasized: Latissimus dorsi, trapezius, biceps, erector spinae, and forearms.

Exercise Technique

1. Start the exercise with your right knee and hand on a bench, back straight and parallel with the floor, dumbbell hanging from your left arm.
2. Point your elbow toward the ceiling as you pull the dumbbell upward.
3. Return the dumbbell to the fully stretched starting position.
4. After completing the requisite number of repetitions, switch the positions, holding the dumbbell in your right hand, and repeat the exercise for the right side of your body.

Training Tip

Stick with dumbbells. Compared to the barbell version of this exercise, a dumbbell allows for a greater range of motion by allowing rotation of the torso during the exercise movement. The result is a greater range of functional strength.

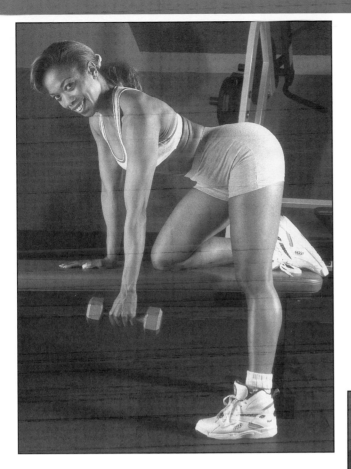

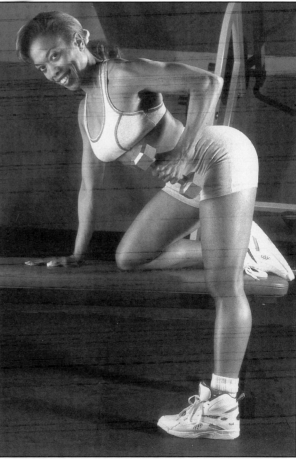

Bent-Over Barbell Row

Muscles Emphasized: Latissimus dorsi, trapezius, erector spinae, biceps, and forearms.

Exercise Technique

1. Start the exercise with your knees slightly bent, bending at the waist, back straight, barbell hanging at arm's length.

2. Keeping the back straight while maintaining the bend in the waist, pull the barbell upward until it touches your torso.

3. Under control, return the barbell to the starting position.

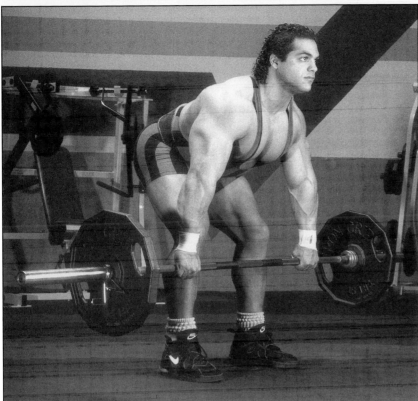

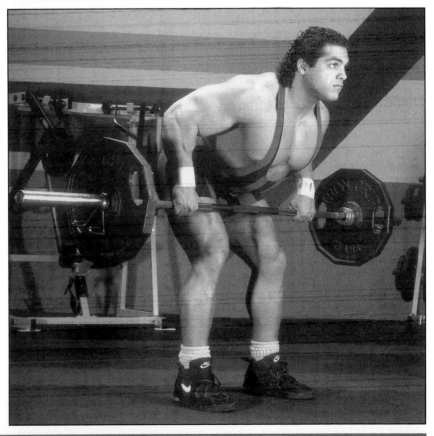

BENT-OVER BARBELL ROW

Seated Long Pull

Muscles Emphasized: Latissimus dorsi, erector spinae, trapezius, biceps, and forearms.

Exercise Technique

1. Start the exercise with your arm, shoulder, and upper back stretched forward to resist the pull of the weight.
2. Pull the handle toward your rib cage as far as possible.
3. Return to the starting position: arms, shoulders, and back stretched forward. That's a rep.

Training Tip

The stimulus of the two-armed long pulls can be varied by changing handles from workout to workout.

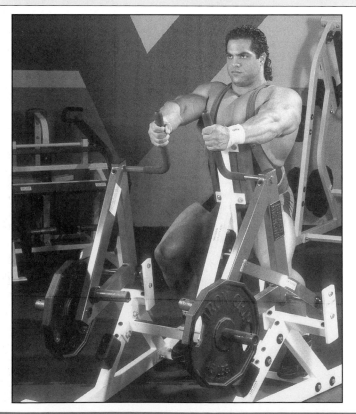

Double-arm pull.

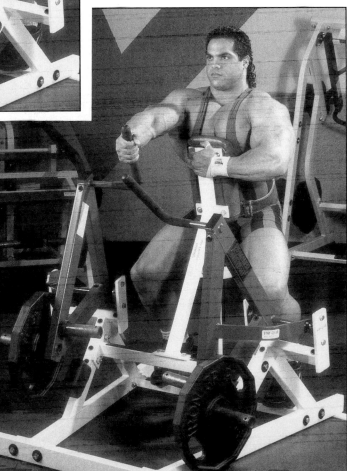

Single-arm pull.

SEATED LONG PULL

Barbell Push Press

Muscles Emphasized: Deltoids, trapezius, erector spinae, triceps, quadriceps

Exercise Technique

1. Feet should be parallel and shoulder-width apart. Pick up bar off rack and place on upper chest.

2. Start the movement by squatting approximately 30 to 40 degrees, with elbows forward and head up. Immediately thrust the legs straight, pushing the barbell upward. Continue the barbell's acceleration by pushing with your arms until your arms are fully extended. Continuous leg-arm thrust is necessary for this explosive sequence.

3. Pause at the top momentarily, then, maintaining control throughout, lower the bar to the starting position at the shoulders. That's a rep.

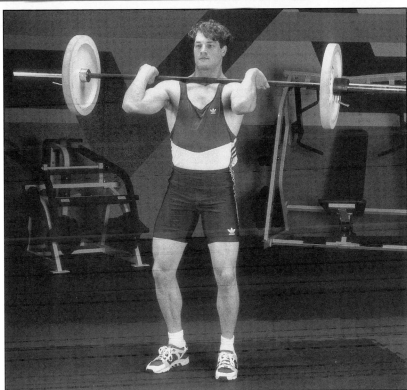

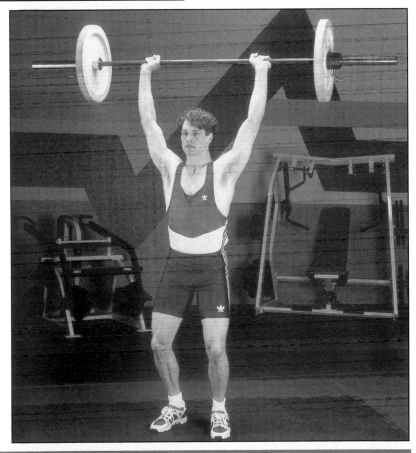

Machine Push Press

An alternative to the barbell push press.

A machine, "The Jammer," is used by many professional and college football teams to duplicate the same sequence of leg drive-shoulder thrust-triceps extension present in the barbell push press.

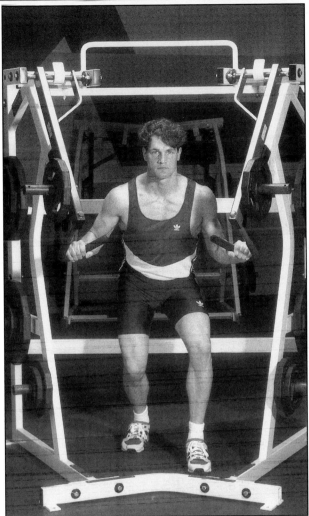

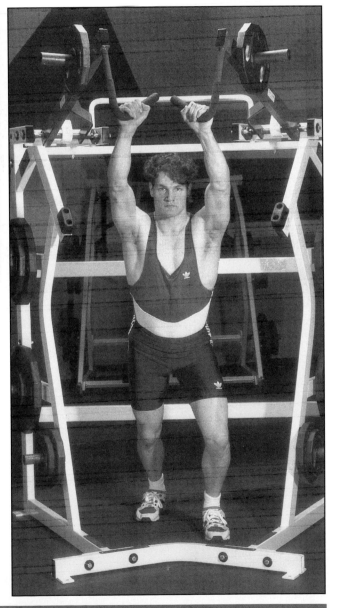

Seated Alternating Overhead Dumbbell Press

Muscles Emphasized: Deltoids and triceps.

Exercise Technique

1. Paying particular attention to stabilizing the lower back, press one dumbbell to arm's length.
2. Lower the dumbbell to the shoulder, simultaneously pressing the opposite dumbbell to arm's length.
3. Lower the second dumbbell and repeat the sequence.

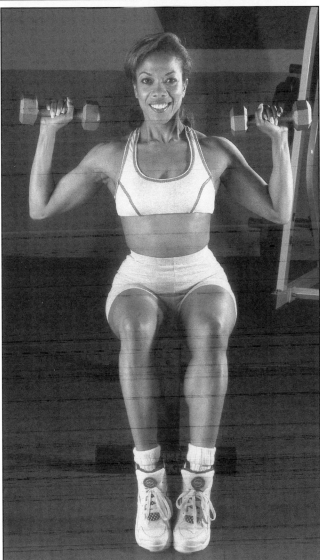

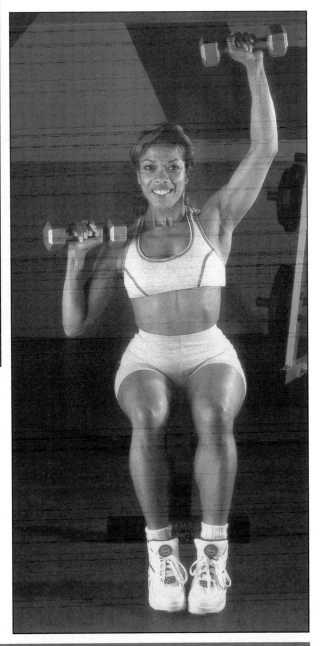

Machine Overhead Press

An alternative to the seated dumbbell press.

Muscles Emphasized: Deltoids and triceps.

Exercise Technique

1. Sit, fasten seat belt, and hold handles above your shoulders.

2. Press handles overhead, together or alternating.

3. Do not arch back.

4. Slowly return to the starting position.

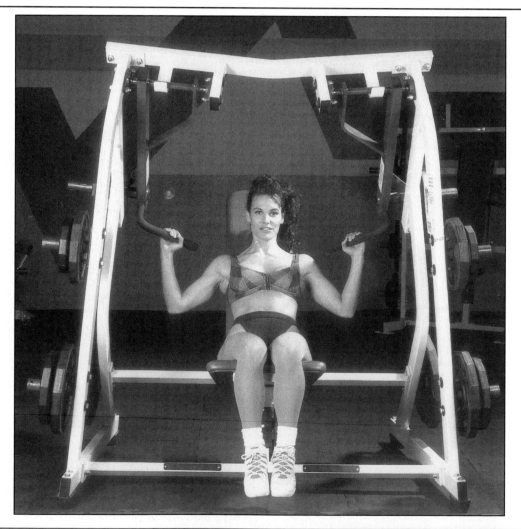

MACHINE OVERHEAD PRESS

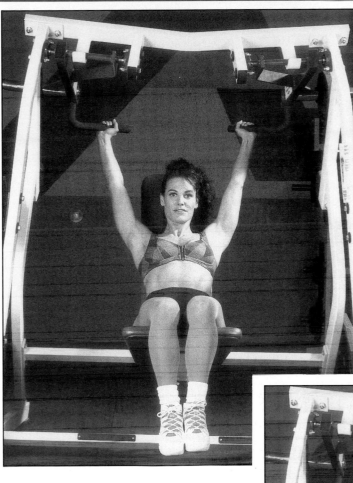

Double-arm press.

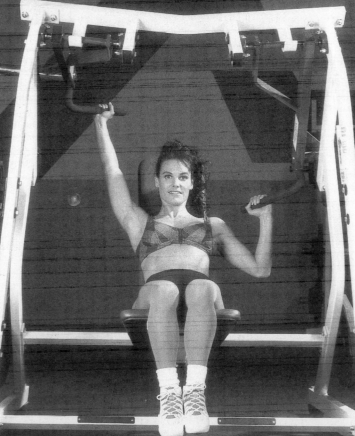

Single-arm press.

MACHINE OVERHEAD PRESS

Alternating Upright Row

Muscles Emphasized: Deltoids, trapezius, biceps, and forearms.

Exercise Technique

1. Stand erect with your feet shoulder width apart, dumbbells hanging at your sides, palms facing your body.

2. Pull the dumbbell up your body, keeping your elbow higher than the dumbbell throughout the movement. At the top of the movement, the natural motion of the pull should find the dumbbell positioned at the front of the shoulder, elbow up.

3. Lower the dumbbell under control to the starting position.

4. Repeat the movement with the opposite arm.

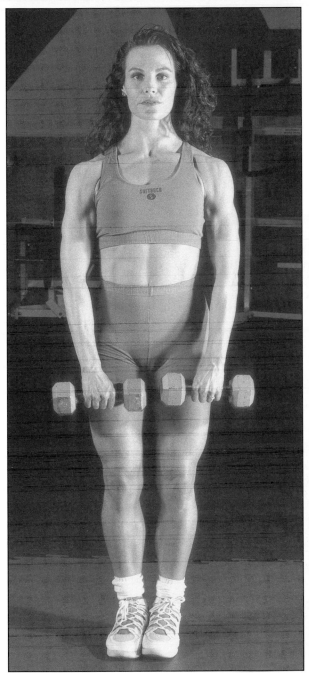

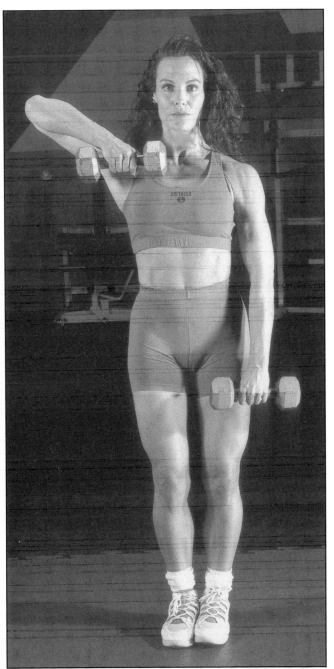

Upright Row

Muscles Emphasized: Deltoids, trapezius, biceps, and forearms.

Exercise Technique

1. Using a barbell or machine, stand erect, feet shoulder width apart, weight hanging at arm's length with an overhand grip.

2. Pull the barbell upward to shoulder height, keeping your elbows higher than the bar at all times. If using a machine, pull bars up until your forearms are parallel to the floor.

3. Lower the weight under control to the starting position.

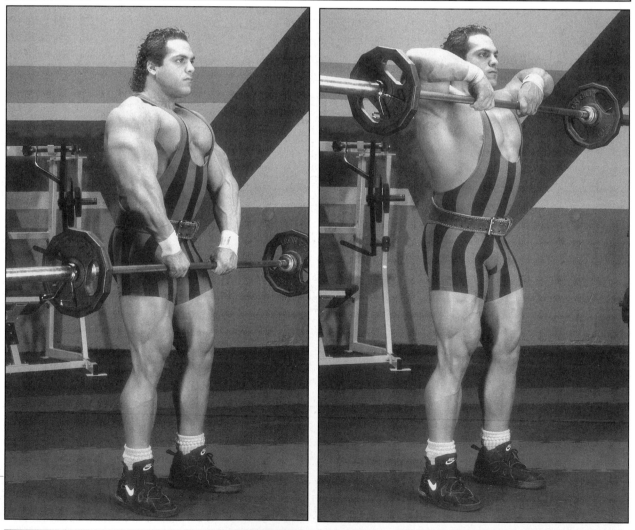

Barbell upright row.

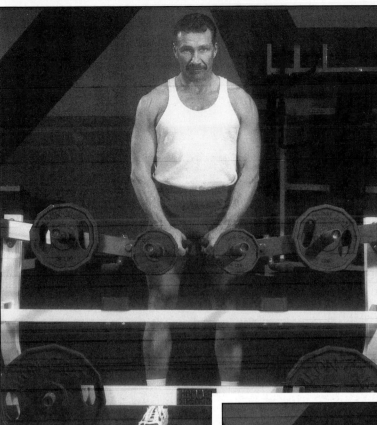

Machine upright row.

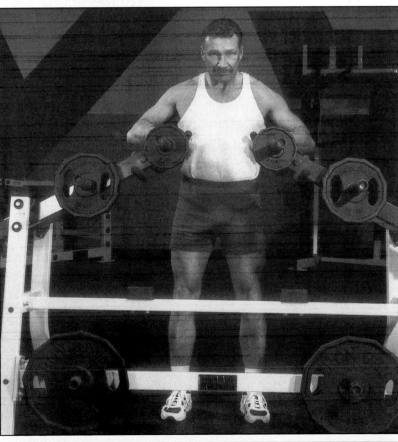

Standing Side Lateral Raises

Muscles Emphasized: Medial deltoids, trapezius, and anterior deltoids.

Exercise Technique

1. Stand erect with feet shoulder width apart. Hold dumbbells or barbell plates with an overhand grip in front of your hips, elbows slightly bent.
2. Raise your arms straight up laterally until your elbows lock and your upper arms are parallel to the floor.
3. Lower your arms to your sides.
4. Repeat the repetitions as required.

Training Tip

Don't swing the dumbbells! Doing so minimizes the resistance at the low point, reducing the effectiveness of the exercise.

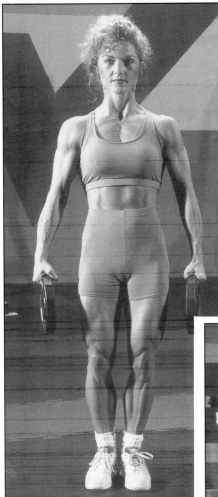

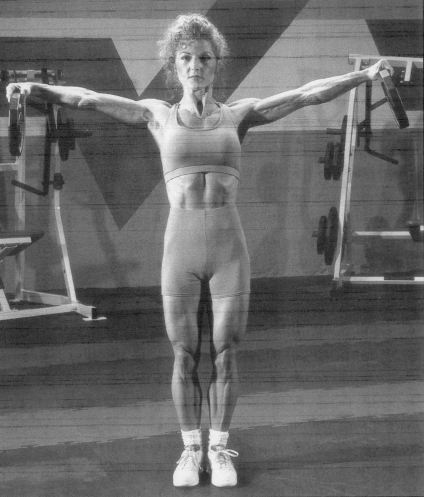

STANDING SIDE LATERAL RAISES

Machine Lateral Raise

An alternative to standing side lateral raises.

Muscles Emphasized: Medial deltoids, trapezius, and anterior deltoids.

Exercise Technique

1. Sit, fasten seat belt, press forearms against the arm pads.
2. Elbows should be slightly behind torso and pressed firmly against pads.
3. Raise elbows slowly to chin level.
4. Return slowly to starting position.

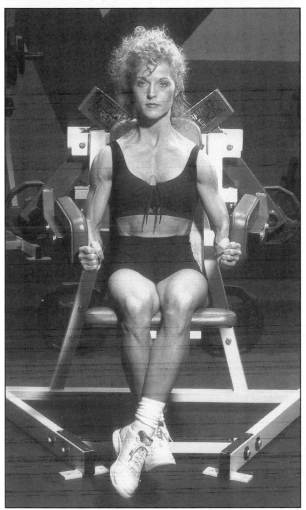

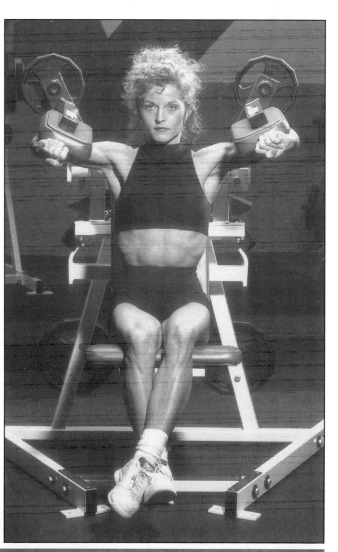

Standing Front Lateral Raises

Muscles Emphasized: Deltoids and trapezius.

Exercise Technique

1. Stand erect with feet shoulder width apart. Hold dumbbells with an overhand grip in front of your hips, elbows slightly bent.

2. Raise your arms straight up in front of your body until your elbows lock and your upper arms are parallel to the floor.

3. Lower your arms to the starting position.

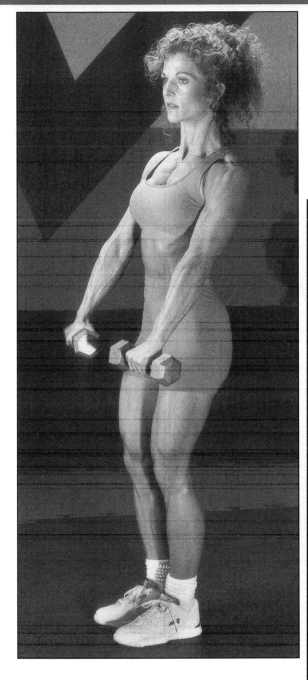

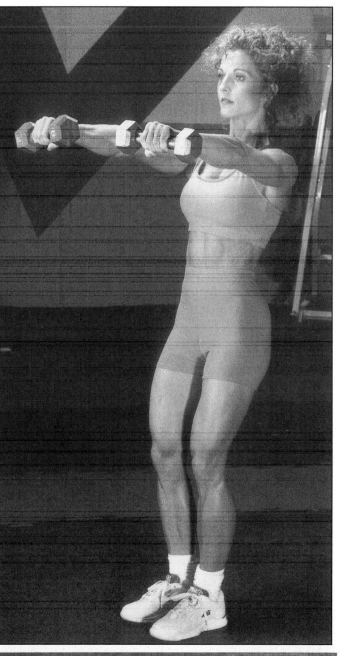

STANDING FRONT LATERAL RAISES

Barbell Biceps Curl

Muscles Emphasized: Biceps and brachialis.

Exercise Technique

1. Standing erect, hang the barbell at arm's length, palms facing away from your body.

2. Without swinging the barbell to enhance acceleration, curl the barbell through a semicircle to your chin. The elbow remains down and the upper arm remains pressed to the body through the movement.

3. Lower the barbell through the same arc. Repeat.

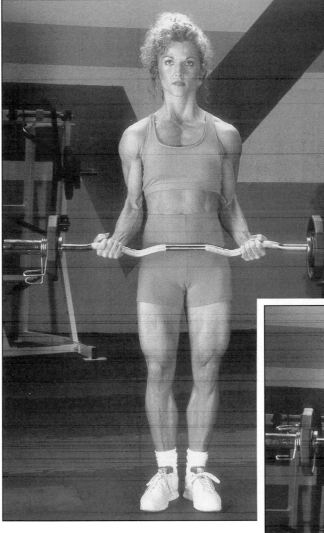

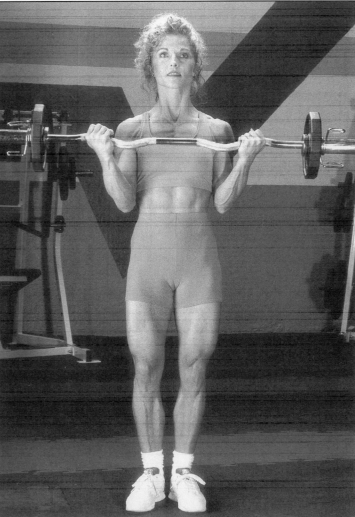

BARBELL BICEPS CURL

Concentration Biceps Curl

Muscles Emphasized: Biceps and brachialis.

Exercise Technique

1. Sit on the end of the bench, holding the dumbbell and positioning the weight between the thighs as pictured. Your upper arm should be braced against the inside of your thigh.

2. As you curl the dumbbell through a semicircle, concentrate on the biceps muscles.

3. Lower the dumbbell. Repeat with the opposite arm.

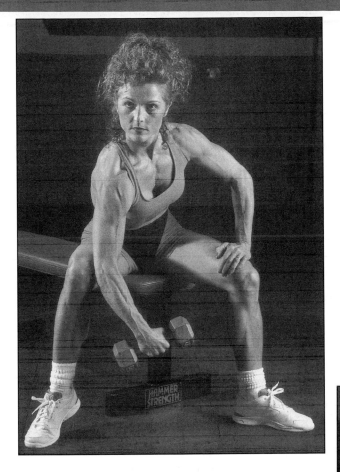

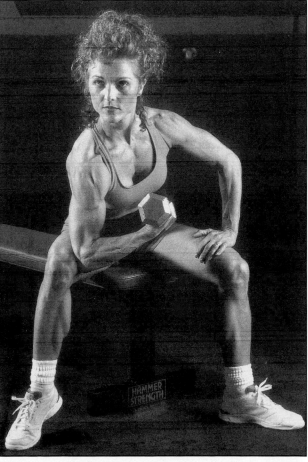

CONCENTRATION BICEPS CURL

Machine Biceps Curl

An alternative to the barbell and concentration curls.

Muscles Emphasized: Biceps and brachialis.

Exercise Technique

1. While seated, grip the handles with an underhand grip, palms facing upward, elbows extended and pressed firmly against the arm pad.
2. Curl one or both hands in an arc toward your chin.
3. Return through the same arc to the starting position.

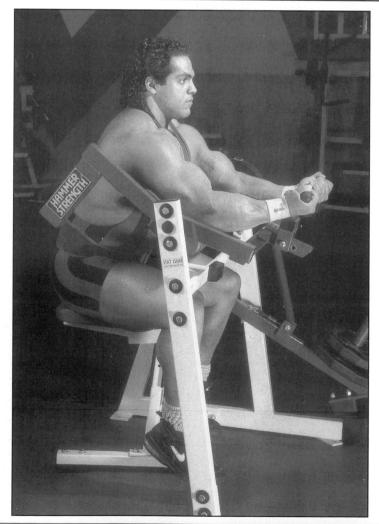

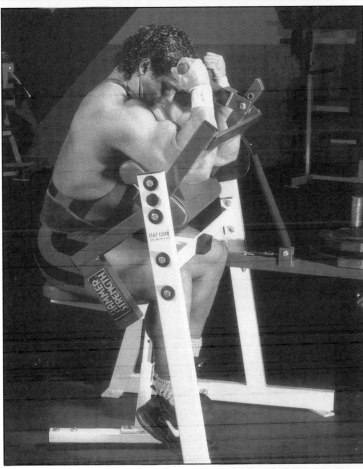

Double-arm curl.

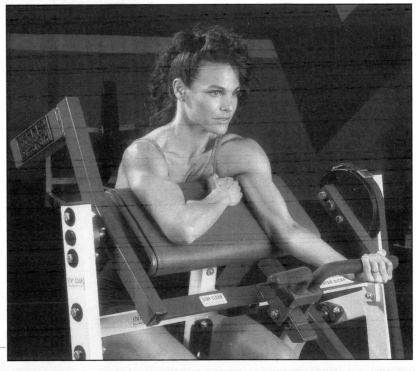

Single-arm curl.

Lying Barbell Triceps Extension

Muscles Emphasized: Triceps.

Exercise Technique

1. Lie on your back. Grip a barbell with your palms up and your hands spaced 6 to 12 inches apart. Hold the barbell at arm's length above your shoulders.

2. Keeping your upper arm perpendicular to your torso, lower the bar through an arc until the backs of your hands touch your forehead.

3. Return the barbell through the arc to the starting position, keeping the upper arm perpendicular to your torso throughout the movement. That's a rep.

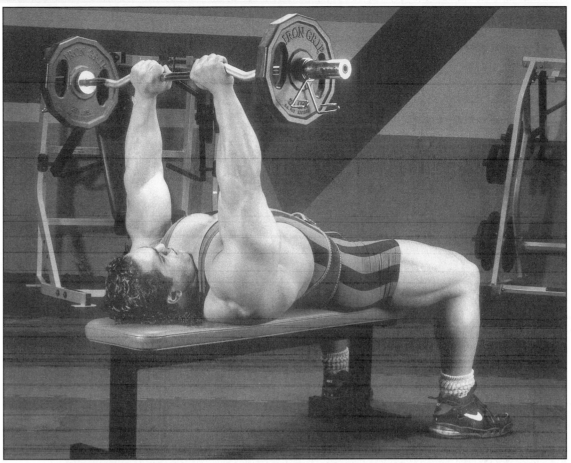

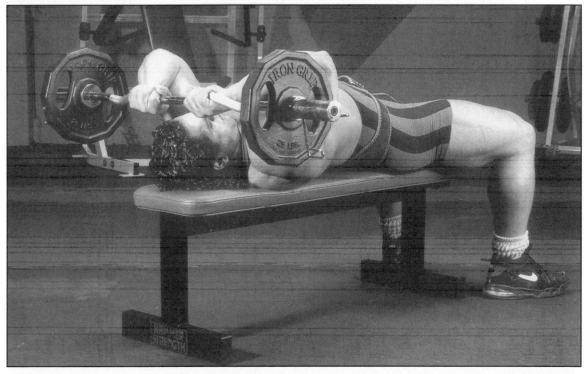

LYING BARBELL TRICEPS EXTENSION

Seated Dumbbell Triceps Extension

Muscles Emphasized: Triceps.

Exercise Technique

1. Hold dumbbell in right hand and raise overhead to arm's length.
2. Sit erect, head up, with your feet on the floor. Keep upper arm close to head.
3. Lower dumbbell in semicircular motion behind your head until your forearm touches your biceps.
4. Return under control to starting position.

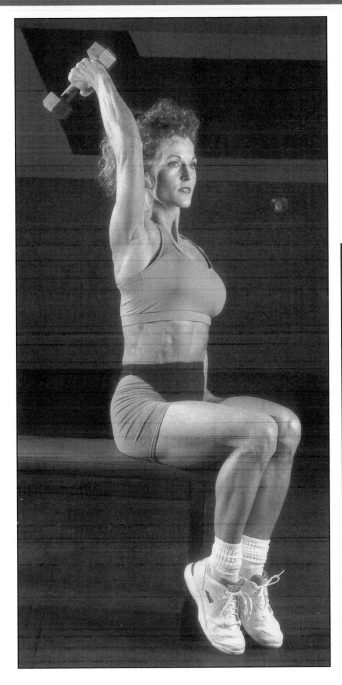

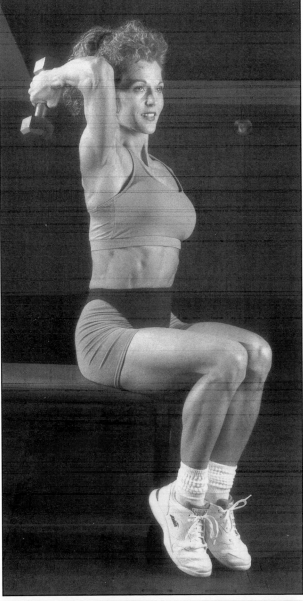

SEATED DUMBBELL TRICEPS EXTENSION

Machine Triceps Extension

An alternative to the seated or lying triceps extension.

Muscles Emphasized: Triceps.

Exercise Technique

1. Sit with arms bent, elbows on pad, and your hands, with palms turned inward, against pads on extension bar.
2. Straighten arms smoothly.
3. Pause, and return slowly to starting position.

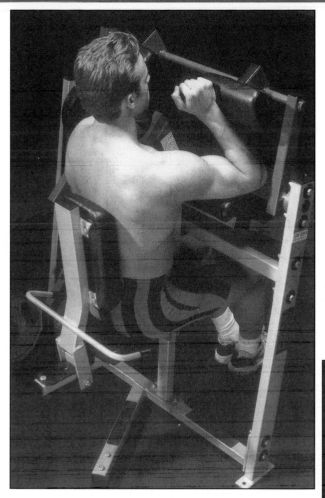

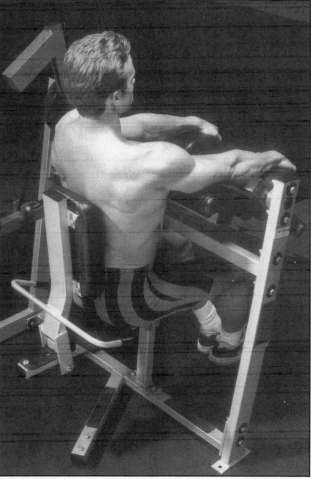

Triceps Kickback

Muscles Emphasized: Triceps and anterior deltoids.

Exercise Technique

1. Place one knee and hand on a bench, and lean forward at the waist. With your free upper arm bent and held close to your body, hold a dumbbell in that hand.

2. While keeping your upper arm parallel with the floor, straighten your arm, lifting the dumbbell upward and backward.

3. Return to the starting position through the same arc, keeping your elbow close in and your upper arm parallel to the floor.

4. Repeat the movement.

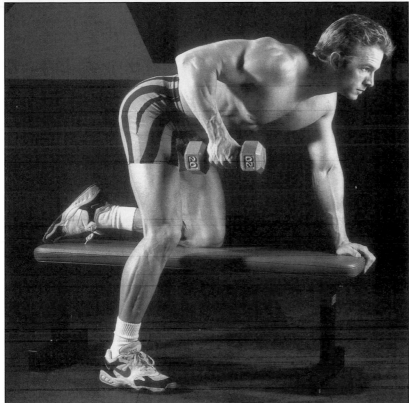

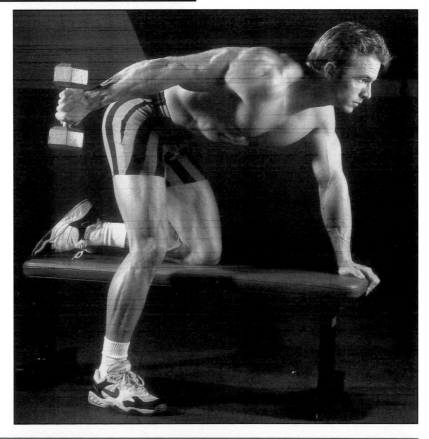

Sit-Ups

Muscles Emphasized: Upper and lower abdominals.

Exercise Technique

1. Lie on a sit-up board inclined to add appropriate resistance with hands clasped behind the neck. If strength permits, hold an appropriately light weighted dumbbell behind the neck to add resistance. Bend your knees.

2. Slowly sit up, keeping your eyes on the ceiling. Pause momentarily after reaching a sitting position.

3. Return slowly to the starting position, concentrating on the abdominals and retaining the bend in the knee throughout the movement. That's a rep.

Training Tip

When training your abdominals, employ the same set and rep pattern as your program requires for any other muscle group. Place a dumbbell behind your neck to increase the resistance when necessary.

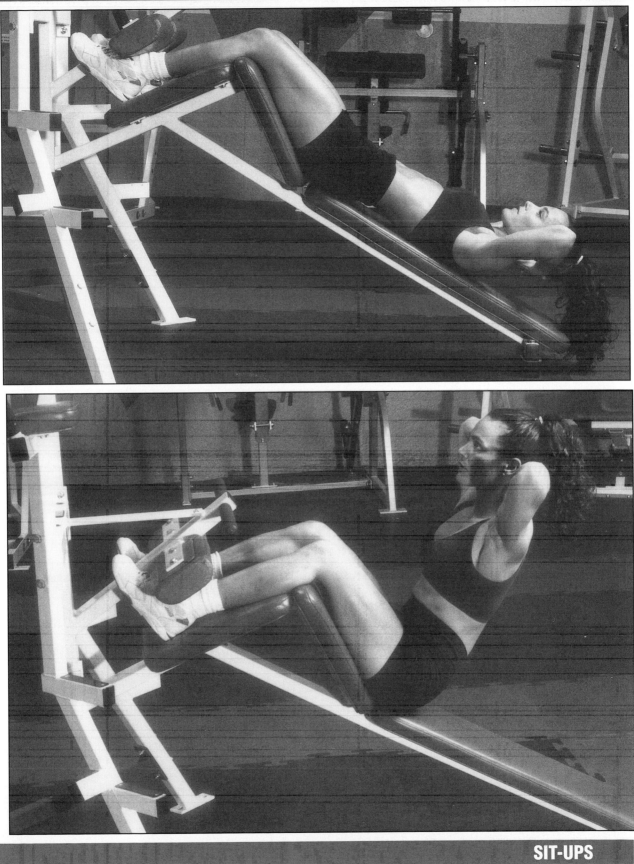

Reverse Trunk Twist

Muscles Emphasized: Abdominals and obliques.

Exercise Technique

1. Lie on your back on the floor, arms extended to your sides for stability, knees bent, and your thighs perpendicular to the floor.
2. Slowly lower your knees to one side of your body, keeping the thighs perpendicular to your torso as your knees touch the floor.
3. Return to the center starting position and lower your thighs to the opposite side.
4. Return to vertical. That's a rep.

Training Tip

This exercise works the muscles responsible for the rotation of the torso. The resistance can be increased by straightening the legs throughout the exercise movement. Add ankle weights for even more resistance.

REVERSE TRUNK TWIST

197

Knee-Ups

Muscles Emphasized: Abdominals and hip flexors.

Exercise Technique

1. To start, support your body weight on elbow pads (or hand from a bar) with your legs extended in line with your body.
2. Raise both knees simultaneously under control, until the thighs are parallel to the floor.
3. Lower the legs to the starting position. That's a rep.

Training Tip

As strength increases, increase the resistance to maintain your set/rep protocol by straightening the legs or adding ankle weights.

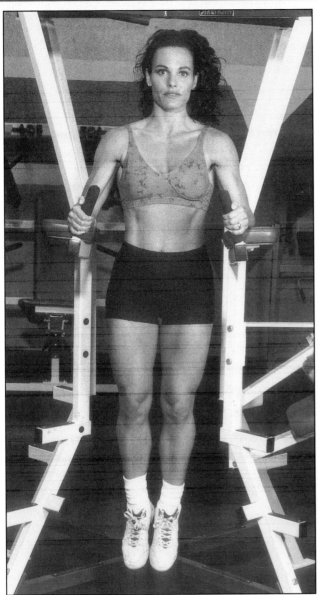

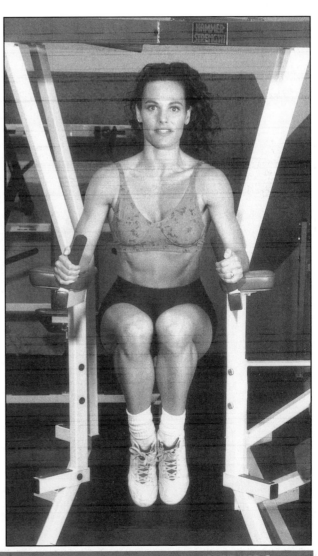

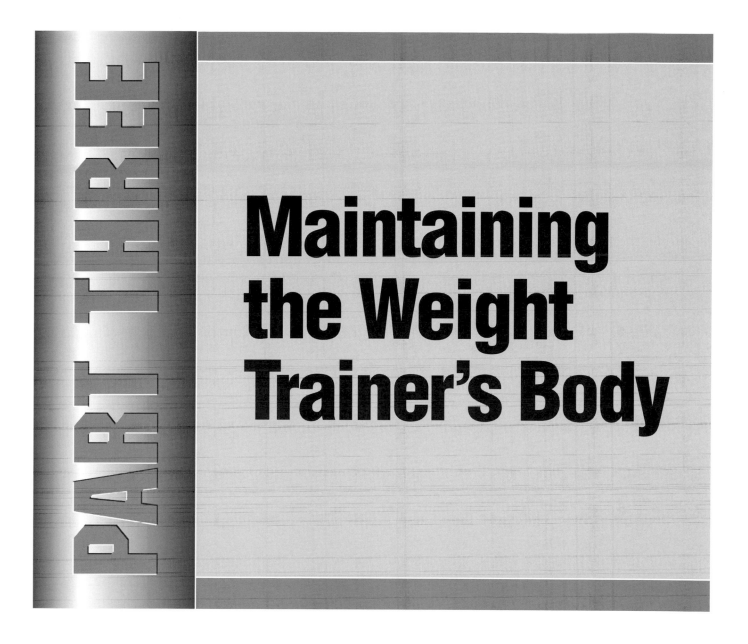

PART THREE

Maintaining the Weight Trainer's Body

Diet, body weight changes, and safety precautions are important factors in planning your overall weight training program. That's because all are factors in meeting your training goals.

Chapter 10, "The Table to Muscle Diet," provides you with the basic nutritional information necessary to develop an adequate, well-balanced training diet. A well-balanced diet is necessary to supply the raw materials for energy production and physical change stimulated by the training demands. Hence, in a real sense, your training goals follow a path from *table to muscle.*

Chapter 11, "Weight Gain, Weight Loss," provides nuts-and-bolts explanations of your body's response to weight change. Weight change, and the corresponding change in energy balance, affect the adaptational capacity of muscle tissue and determine whether a weight training program will build or destroy muscle tissue. Clearly, the muscles' response to a change in body weight is an important topic to consider in light of your training goals.

Chapter 12, "Training Safely and Nursing Injuries," opens with rules for safe training that are designed to protect you from injury during your weight training experience. Although rare and usually minor, injuries do happen. Chapter 12 offers suggestions for treating those unavoidable injuries.

Although you're on the final leg of the book, treat the material in the following chapters as importantly as you do the exercise programs that precede them. Meeting your training goals requires a comprehensive program, both in and outside the gymnasium.

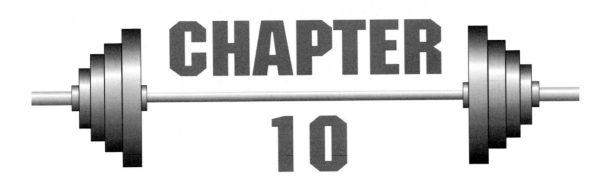

CHAPTER 10

The Table to Muscle Diet

The saying, "You are what you eat," is true. Of course, that means some people probably have the body chemistry of jelly doughnuts. What you eat also partly defines what you are able to do. Fruit juice, protein power bars, crepes suzette, hamburgers—all foods supply energy and nutrients. The weight trainer's concern is eating foods that have enough energy and the right balance of nutrients to facilitate her lifting a weight, serving an ace, or paddling a canoe through the rapids.

If we were talking mechanical equipment, we would point out that only the best high-test fuel is pumped into Indianapolis 500 race cars. It should be no different for the finely tuned human being at the wheel. That brings us to an important point: Foods differ drastically in the amount of energy they supply, the speed with which they supply it, and the nutrients contained therein. Like people, foods have different attributes. Knowing the full range of a particular food's attributes provides you with the information to make an intelligent choice to select those foods that will help you reach your weight training goals.

Every person should be careful about diet. An athlete's energy requirements will vary due to body weight, height, age, sex, metabolic rate, and the type, intensity, and duration of the sport. In fact, the best diet for an active athlete is not much different than for a sedentary accountant. However, training frequency and competition do make some extra demands, which we will discuss in this section. We'll serve up foods according to their components: protein, fat, carbohydrates, vitamins, minerals, and water. All are not only important but *essential* to life.

Just eating all those different components isn't enough. They must be eaten in the right proportions, in what is called a *well-balanced diet*. That doesn't mean three trays per day filled with a Big Mac, fries, and Coke—balanced with a fruit pie for dessert. The accepted meaning of a well-balanced diet is our first stop on the path of basic nutrition knowledge.

WELL-BALANCED: A LITTLE OF EVERYTHING

There's nothing wrong with a Big Mac, fries, and Coke in spite of the cacophony of babble from the high priests of a fat-conscious society. Nevertheless, you don't want to eat exclusively off a fast-food menu. In practice, balance means disciplining yourself to eat enough of everything, but not too much of any one thing.

Balance is the operative word in an important concept, *balance of foodstuffs*. That's what you need. A balance of vitamins and minerals. A balance of proteins, fats, and carbohydrates. A balance between nutrients found in juices and Cokes. To meet your weight training goals, your dietary goal is to create a gastronomic stew from a recipe containing the broadest possible base of ingredients—in the right balance—to meet your body's needs.

Through decades of political and scientific input, the governmental agency responsible for dietary information, the USDA, has established statistics-based recommendations for a well-balanced diet. Those recommendations are graphically explained in figure 10.1. The foundation of the pyramid represents the foods to be eaten most, and the peak of that pyramid represents the foods to be eaten least. A quick glance at the pyramid can help you decide if you're statistically on the recommended nutritional track.

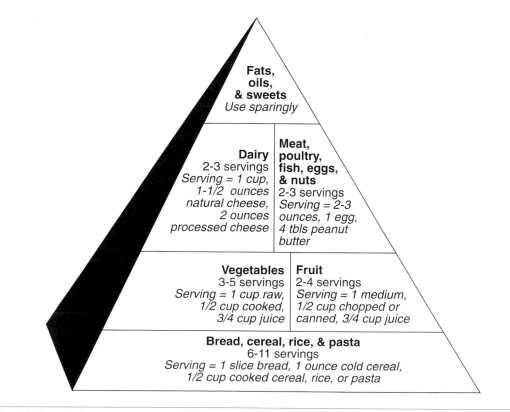

Fig. 10.1. The base of the USDA food pyramid represents the foods to be eaten most to satisfy energy requirements. Foods to be eaten least are found at the top of the pyramid.

Data from the U.S. Department of Agriculture/U.S. Department of Health and Human Services.

A Well-Balanced Diet Is a Personal Thing

Now, what about *you*? Your diet is well-balanced if it supplies you with the nutrients to meet *your* nutritional needs. That includes enough energy to supply your energy expenditures and enough nutrients to repair old tissue and build new tissue.

Nutritionists have quantified the "right balance" of foods for the *statistically average* person. In fact, they've broken that balance into basic ingredients of fats, carbohydrates, and proteins. Under those terms, a well-balanced diet has the following proportion of raw ingredients:

◆ 15% protein;

◆ 60% carbohydrate; and

◆ 25% fat.

For the nutritionist's hypothetical person, consuming 1,800 calories per day to meet her energy demands, about 70 grams of protein, 270 grams of carbohydrates, and 50 grams of fat satisfy the recommendations.

However, the recommended proportions appear absurd when discussing inordinately active people. For example, a weightlifter or marathoner having triple the average person's daily energy needs—5,400 calories—would require more than 200 grams of protein, 800 grams of carbohydrates, and 150 grams of fat to satisfy the recommendations. That's a lot of fat to clog the intestine and a lot of protein waste product to be metabolized through the liver.

The point being made is that the statistically correct, well-balanced diet is inherently arbitrary when applied to individual cases that stray from the statistical center. *You* are probably one of those cases if you're a high-performance athlete, aerobic dancer, or intense weight trainer.

What can you do? Unfortunately, there is no one answer. You're going to have to experiment to find your best balance of fats, carbohydrates, and proteins. But a word of caution is in order: Don't stray too far from the general recommendations without the input of expert advice. One definite mistake is to follow the dietary fads of a bodybuilding magazine.

Proceed with caution, and do your best to make reasonable choices. Discuss your personal training needs with medical and training experts, and read on.

The Rationale for a Balanced Diet

Here's a short but pointed list of reasons why it's so important that you meet your energy needs through a balance of nutrients.

◆ **Proteins** are absolutely necessary to maintain and build *every* nerve cell, muscle cell, and bone cell in your body. Rather than grow, muscle would be destroyed with too little protein consumption.

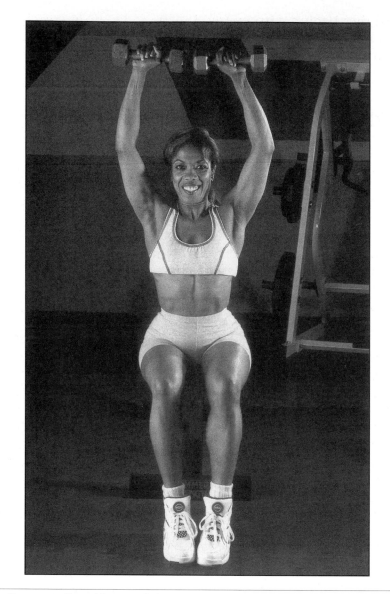

Every muscle cell, nerve cell, and bone cell depends on a well-balanced diet for optimal maintenance and growth.

◆ **Carbohydrates** are a muscle cell's main source of energy, the fuel that energizes protein utilization. Too little carbohydrate, even with adequate protein, produces a net loss of muscle tissue.

◆ **Fats**—two of which are essential to life—are part of every cell. Storing essential, fat soluble vitamins requires fat in the diet.

◆ **Vitamins** are the cell's catalysts: A deficiency of any one vitamin will impede or stop cell functions, leading to a loss in performance, or death.

◆ **Minerals** are absolutely necessary for enzyme and hormone production and cell formation and maintenance.

That's a short list of the thousands of reasons that a well-balanced diet is an absolute necessity for the weight trainer who wants to maximize the results of his training program.

A balanced diet begins with energy balance, which is simply making sure that energy consumption equals energy expenditure. Keeping tabs on energy means counting calories.

COUNTING CALORIES

Different measurements of the weight trainer's body require different units: height in feet and inches, weight in pounds; familiar, easily understood units relative to everyday experience. The weight trainer's energy is measured in less tangible units—calories. Most people know of calories in connection with diets; usually only in terms of guilt or something Rocky Road ice cream has in excess. However, we can't use a yardstick or a scale to measure them.

Calories are nondiscriminatory. A calorie from the fat in Rocky Road ice cream is the same amount of energy as a calorie from pure protein. And whether marathoners or couch potatoes, we measure the available energy in the food we eat in terms of calories.

Ounce per ounce, or gram per gram, foodstuffs differ in amounts of energy (calories) they provide. A piece of chocolate cream pie can be converted into hundreds of energy-equivalent calories, but water, on the other hand, provides us with none, because the body can't convert water—even hot water—into usable energy.

In a laboratory, the number of calories available from an apple, an orange, or a piece of pie is determined by measuring the amount of heat it takes to completely burn them. The constituent ingredients of common foods can be determined, too. The caloric values of carbohydrates, fats, and proteins are:

> ### GETTING SPECIFIC: HOW THE FOOD AND DRUG ADMINISTRATION DEFINES CALORIE
>
> Given the latest range of food products available to calorie-conscious consumers, perhaps you've wondered what the different usage of calorie means. Here are the Food and Drug Administration definitions:
>
> **Calorie free:** fewer than 5 calories per serving
>
> **Low calorie:** 40 calories or less per serving; if the serving is 30 grams or less or 2 tablespoons or less, per 50 grams of the food
>
> **Reduced or fewer calories:** at least 25 percent fewer calories per serving than reference food (for example, reduced calorie ice cream must have 25% fewer calories than regular ice cream)

- ◆ 1 gram of carbohydrate = 4 calories (1 ounce = 114 calories)
- ◆ 1 gram of fat = 9 calories (1 ounce = 255 calories)
- ◆ 1 gram of protein = 4 calories (1 ounce = 114 calories)

(By the way, 454 grams equal 1 pound. Hence, a gram cracker is much smaller than a graham cracker.)

Fortunately, you don't need a lab to check the various calorie contents of food; Just get a "calorie counter," a booklet containing a food-by-food evaluation of calorie content. You can find these for less than a dollar at most supermarkets. It's one of the easiest ways to check.

"Empty calories" is a pop-culture term referring to foods that have calories with little additional nutritional value. In other words, they're out of balance: lots of calories but little of the other ingredients—the basic nutrients—necessary to sustain a healthy body. The next section describes those basic nutrients.

BASIC NUTRIENTS

Snails in garlic butter. Banana-cream cake. Asparagus in hollandaise sauce. Liver and onions. All the disparate foods we eat can be broken down into six distinguishable groups, each of which has special qualities that satisfy different body needs. Water, proteins, fats, carbohydrates, vitamins, and minerals are collectively called the basic nutrients.

The basic nutrients have three jobs: supply energy, sustain tissue growth and repair, and catalyze or otherwise participate in thousands of life-supporting chemical reactions—in fact, *all* life-supporting chemical reactions.

These next few sections explore the body's dependence on basic nutrients. We'll begin with the body's most common nutrient, water.

HOW MUCH WATER SHOULD YOU DRINK?

The best advice: Drink when in doubt! More water is better than less water. Recommending an ideal amount for *you* isn't any more possible than recommending your ideal calorie consumption without knowing your weight, the climate, your training program, and so on. As a rule of thumb, I can recommend that you drink throughout the day, continuous small drinks, never chancing the potential for temporary dehydration. Try to drink at least six to eight 8-ounce glasses of water a day and, of course, drink more when training hard or in hot weather.

You're All Wet!

More than 70 percent of your adult fat-free body is plain old water. It's a good thing, too, because even though water has no calories, vitamins, minerals, or usable energy, it is second only to oxygen as the most required substance. Without a continuous supply of it, we would quickly—as it were—kick the bucket.

Most (about two-thirds) of your body's water is located inside your cells, in varying proportions depending on the type of cell. You can think of the cells as containing a conglomerate of chemical structures floating in a water-based liquid. It's a wonder we don't slosh when we move.

After cells, blood is the champion water glutton. The average weight trainer has about a gallon of water as blood fluid. Floating along in this stream of water are the oxygen-carrying red blood cells and lots of proteins, fats, carbohydrates, vitamins, and minerals that must be delivered to the cells. Water is also an essential contributor to the body's cooling and nervous systems and acts as a safety cushion to the spinal cord, joints, and brain. It's instrumental in every body function.

Humans derive water from three general sources. The most obvious is the liquids we drink; the milk, coffee, juices, and sodas. When we feel our water content running low, we reach for a drink to satisfy our immediate thirst. Food is also an important source of water. Of course, some foods are better water sources than others. A soda cracker has less than 5% water content. That's one reason it's an excellent food to soak up the acids of an upset stomach. On the other hand, a stalk of celery is more than 90% water. That's one reason it's an excellent diet food.

A third source of water is energy metabolism. As carbohydrates, fats, and proteins are metabolized to provide cellular energy, varying amounts of water are released into the system. Those of you who took high school biology may recall that water-releasing reactions are condensation reactions.

In just a few hours of intense training in hot weather, an athlete can easily lose 5 percent of his or her body's water. Even the Sedentary Sams and Couch Potato Pams lose substantial amounts through evaporation and urination—so much that they would die in several days without replenishing the supply with a little gulp here and a little gulp there.

Little gulps of water should be ingested before, during, and after exercise. Gulping down huge amounts at one time won't do anything but bloat the stomach. That's because the bloodstream can only absorb about a quart per hour, so the best method is to take small but frequent drinks.

When the body is extremely low on water, *every* system and *every* cell is affected: the cooling system falters and the body temperature rises; the blood thickens, causing the circulatory system to malfunction; elimination of waste through urination is inhibited; and nervous impulses go haywire. The weight trainer's strength, coordination, and overall performance break down. The point to all this is simply put: Water's cheap; drink it often.

Protein Is No Panacea

Since the earliest days of weight training, weight lifters believed that muscle wouldn't substantially grow without relatively huge quantities of protein. Scientific studies have generally shown that weight trainers probably need little more protein than law clerks or mattress testers—60 to 70 grams a day for an average-size mattress tester (160 pounds). Decades of weight lifters and bodybuilders ate enormous quantities of protein, thinking the increased protein necessary for increased muscle mass. Extra protein, yes, but not an enormous increase over average amounts. Recommendation: As insurance, the strength athlete should consume three-fourths of a gram of protein for every pound of body weight—that's 50% more than the recommended amount for the nonathlete.

The early weight trainers were hooked by a little information—muscle cells contain protein—and the outrageous claims of magazine publishers (who sold protein powders). Rest assured that if your foods contain 15% protein, you're getting enough.

Notwithstanding the above, adequate protein consumption is absolutely necessary for a successful weight training program. Digestion breaks that raw protein into its constituent amino acids. In turn, the amino acids are the basic building blocks of muscle growth. Twenty-two different amino acids are needed by the cell for proper maintenance and growth. Your body can actually manufacture 14 of these needed amino acids from constituent parts found in a normal diet. The other eight amino acids, called the essential amino acids, can't be manufactured from raw materials; they must be continually obtained from protein-laden foods. Since amino acids can't be stored in the liver, lungs, lymph glands, or anywhere else from head to toe, they must be eaten on a daily basis.

The raw proteins contained in foods are classified as either complete or incomplete. A complete protein is one that has all eight essential amino acids. An incomplete protein is one that lacks one or more of the essentials. Common sources of complete protein are meat, eggs, and milk. Few plants contain complete proteins, but that's not a problem, even for vegetarians, because all the essential amino acids *don't* have to come from the same food source. The important factor is that the total food intake supplies the essentials. Peanuts and peas, while not being complete proteins in themselves, combine to supply all eight essential amino acids. Once combined in the digestive system, the original source doesn't matter.

A protein deficiency is rare in industrialized countries. Considering that a quart of milk contains 32 grams of complete protein, you can see how easy it is to get a day's supply of 60 to 70 grams.

One last point. The weight trainer can get too much protein, and too much can cause physical problems by overworking the liver and kidneys. Once again, the best advice can be summed up in one word: balance!

PROTEIN SUPPLEMENTS?

Athletes are bombarded by advertisements on the latest food fads that promise improved physical performance and appearance, and many of them are taken to the cleaners—not to a higher training plateau—by buying prepackaged protein and amino acid drinks, powders, or pills, which can cost in excess of $50 per pound of protein. In addition, protein supplements may be derived from poor-quality protein sources and often must be blended with milk, a high-quality protein (which is readily available and cheaper) in order to make them nutritionally complete.

Intake of these new "designer protein" supplements can add as little as one gram of protein to an athlete's diet to more than 100 to 200 grams per day. Research indicates that protein intake in excess of two to three times the RDA has not been shown to enhance physical endurance or muscle strength.

A Love Note to Lard

Don't let the word "fat" scare you. You need fat in your diet *and* on your hips to stay healthy, energetic, and warm.

All foods contain fat, varying from less than 1% in most fruits and vegetables to 100% in lard. A hamburger and fries falls near the middle.

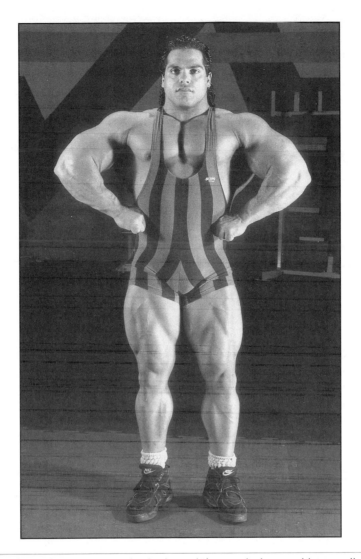

It takes a lot of calories to fuel a large, active body, and those calories need be supplied through a well-balanced diet to provide adequate nutrients for maintenance and growth.

Fats in our diet, we know, add flavor and texture and satisfy our hunger. Fats are highly concentrated energy sources; more than 4,200 calories per pound, compared to about 1,700 calories for a pound of carbohydrates. Fats also provide more than twice as many calories as protein.

Energy production differences are even more significant when comparing stored fats (fat cells) and carbohydrates: 1 pound of body fat stores as much usable energy as 14 pounds of carbohydrates. That's a 3,500 to 250 per pound calorie advantage. Considering the relative disparity in energy production, you can quickly understand the selective advantage in our evolutionary ancestors developing big hips rather than big livers.

Each gram of fat has 9 calories—that's equivalent to 255 calories per ounce. The USDA recommends that you limit fat in your diet to 30% of the total calories consumed. There are two types of fat substitutes that are used to give reduced-fat foods the texture, appearance, and taste of full-fat products: carbohydrate-based and protein-based.

Carbohydrate-based fat substitutes, such as modified starches, dextrin, cellulose, and gums, work by combining with water to provide a thicker texture and appearance, as in fat-free salad dressings.

Protein-based fat substitutes, made of skim milk protein, provide the sensation of creaminess as well as improving appearance and texture. Low-fat cheese made with a protein-based substitute has an appearance and texture close to full-fat cheese.

Both types of fat substitutes contribute some calories, although less than are contributed by fat. Often, a combination of ingredients is used to create higher-quality reduced-fat products. As the food industry learns more about using fat substitutes in different foods, we can expect to see more good-tasting, reduced-fat products, such as new brands of baked goods and frozen desserts.

For the dieters among us, it's unfortunate that fat needn't be eaten to be stored. Nearly everything digested—from the carbohydrates in cantaloupe to the protein in cashew nuts—can be converted and stored as fat. The long and short of it is that excess calories—calories remaining after energy expenditures are complete—are converted into fat.

An interesting sidebar is that fat cells are in constant flux; they don't just hang around. Each week, about half the body's fat is replaced as it becomes involved in various metabolic processes from energy production to vitamin transport, but the absolute quantity of fat remains the same unless the calorie balance of ingested food is changed.

Along with energy production, body fat also acts as a living shield, protecting vital organs from impact damage. A kidney or liver could be severely injured during a football game or boxing match if the organ weren't surrounded by a fat cushion. Subcutaneous fat—suet just under the skin—also acts as a living thermal shield, a protective insulation against the cold environment.

One final, important point links dietary fats and fat soluble vitamins. Without dietary fats, vitamins A, D, E, and K could not be absorbed, stored, and used by the body. These essential vitamins can't ride a water molecule to

---

GETTING SPECIFIC: WHAT ARE THE MEASURES OF FAT?

Have you gone shopping for salad dressing and been puzzled by the labels that claim to be low, free, or reduced fat? Are there specific, measured differences to these names? To help clear the confusion, the *Code of Federal Regulations* offers the following definitions of these terms:

Fat free: less than 0.5 gram of fat per serving

Saturated fat free: less than 0.5 gram per serving and the level of trans fatty acids does not exceed 1% of total fat

Low fat: 3 grams or less per serving, and if the serving is 30 grams or less or 2 tablespoons or less, per 50 grams of the food

Low saturated fat: 1 gram or less per serving and not more than 15% of calories from saturated fatty acids

Reduced or less fat: at least 25% less per serving than reference food

Reduced or less saturated fat: at least 25% less per serving than reference food

fulfill their important physiological functions. Hence, a no-fat diet can conceivably lead to vitamin deficiencies.

If fats are so wonderful, why do we need carbohydrates? Since fat-laden foods take longer than carbohydrate foods to convert to usable energy, weight trainers rely on carbohydrates for an immediate energy source. Carbohydrates are the subject of our next section.

Carbohydrates for Quick Energy

Although not as energy-productive as dietary or stored fats, carbohydrates are the primary source of food energy for human beings. In other words, most of the average person's energy needs are satisfied by carbohydrates.

Chemically speaking, let it suffice that carbohydrates are complicated mixtures of hydrogen, oxygen, and carbon. Gastronomically speaking, tangerines, dried figs, and French bread are loaded with carbohydrates, which are composed of the starches and sugars found in plants. The process through which the body converts carbohydrates into energy—a highly complex subject—is simplified in the following paragraphs.

Carbohydrates are classified into three categories: monosaccharides, disaccharides, and polysaccharides. *Saccharide* essentially means sugar molecule. The prefixes, *mono, di,* and *poly* let the reader know the number of sugar molecules in the carbohydrate—meaning one, two, and three or more, respectively.

Here's the sweet spot. *Only* monosaccharides (single sugar molecules) can pass from the intestine into the bloodstream. But worry not, because digestion breaks down most di's and poly's into mono's for use by the body. Hence a nonusable disaccharide (two molecules of sugar bound together) are digested into two monosaccharides that are usable by the body. Complex carbohydrates, such as breads, cereals, rice, and pasta, not only provide energy, but are also low in fat.

Some complex carbohydrates, long strings of sugar molecules (polysaccharides), are too complex in structure to be broken down by the human digestive system. If they can't be broken down into single molecules, they can't pass from the intestine into the bloodstream.

These nondigestible carbohydrates—such as lettuce and celery—retain their carbohydrates and calories, passing through the digestive tract as roughage. That's why they're excellent diet foods.

Monosaccharides are further classified as glucose, fructose, and galactose, each of which is capable of passing from the intestines into the bloodstream. Once entering the bloodstream, glucose is the body's most readily usable energy source. Its particular chemical structure facilitates immediate use at the point of energy demand. That's why eating a candy bar or a spoonful of honey yields quick energy—it's the high glucose content.

Before satisfying an energy need, the other two mono's (fructose and galactose) must make an intermediate stop at the liver, where they are first converted into the more usable glucose. This manufactured glucose is then "liverated" into the bloodstream to find a cell in need. If not immediately needed, it is stored in the liver or muscle as glycogen.

It's important that carbohydrates be included in the daily diet, mostly because the body doesn't store more than a couple of pounds, and a couple of pounds won't go far in a weight trainer's life.

What happens to the weight trainer without a moderate supply of carbohydrates? He or she won't gain strength or muscle. One reason is that carbohydrates regulate protein metabolism; in other words, they must be present to allow the body to assimilate protein for building and repairing the muscles. Another reason is that carbohydrate depletion drains motivation: The brain, unable to store carbohydrates, depends on the bloodstream to deliver a steady stream of glucose for energy. The psychological ramifications of a brain without adequate energy are evident across the spectrum from the demeanor of malnourished children to crash dieters.

By now, I suspect it's obvious why carbohydrates are considered basic nutrients in a well-balanced diet. Considering how easily they are obtained from food, there's no need to go without an adequate supply.

We go next to vitamins—little doses that do a big job.

GETTING SPECIFIC: FDA DEFINITIONS OF SUGAR

Here are the Food and Drug Administration's definitions of "sugar":

Sugar free: less than 0.5 grams per serving

No added sugar, without added sugar, no sugar added:

1. No sugars added during processing or packing, including ingredients that contain sugars (for example, fruit juices, applesauce, or dried fruit).

2. Processing does not increase the sugar content above the amount naturally present in the ingredients. (A functionally insignificant increase in sugars is acceptable from processes used for purposes other than increasing sugar content.)

3. The food that it resembles and for which it substitutes normally contains added sugars.

4. If the food doesn't meet the requirements for a low- or reduced-calorie food, the product bears a statement that the food is not low-calorie or calorie-reduced and directs consumers' attention to the nutrition panel for further information on sugars and calorie content.

Reduced sugar: at least 25% less sugar per serving than reference food

Use Vitamins for Vitality, But Don't Overdose

The word *vitamin* comes from the Latin word for life, which is appropriate since life would be impossible without those invisible organic substances. All foods contain vitamins, but no single food has them all, which is another reason the weight trainer is in need of a well-balanced diet. Vitamins are categorized as either fat-soluble or water-soluble. That is, some need to combine with fat in order to carry out their duties and others need to swim, so to speak, in water. Even to make it from the intestine into the bloodstream, they must travel with the proper partner.

Chances are that missing a few days' supply of fat-soluble vitamins (A, D, E, and K) won't hurt you, because those are stored in the body's fat cells and can be withdrawn from storage if needed.

Ingesting excessive quantities of fat-soluble vitamins can be toxic, particularly to the liver. Lots of well-intentioned weight trainers have done themselves more harm than good by wolfing down megadoses of vitamin supplements like so many gumdrops. The symptoms of this "vitamin poisoning" are sluggishness and indigestion, which aren't likely to help your workouts.

Water-soluble vitamins aren't stored; take too many, and they're harmlessly washed away with urine. But lack of storage is a double edged sword: The weight trainer needs a daily supply, without which his or her performance is hurt in very tangible ways. For instance, not enough B-complex vitamins lowers the speed of nerve impulses and produces cramps, muscular fatigue, loss of concentration, and high blood pressure. That's one reason why many health experts recommend a daily pill containing the water-solubles.

The point to remember about vitamins: A well-balanced diet should supply you with all the vitamins you need, but for added insurance, take a moderate dosage (not a megadosage), multiple vitamin-mineral tablet each day.

Minerals: Eat Your Chromium

Superman is the Man of Steel, but the rest of us can brag that, at least in part, we're made of chromium, with magnesium muscles and iron blood cells. We don't clank when we walk or turn green from corrosion, but the minerals needed by the body are the same ones taken from the ground to manufacture automobiles, pipe, and refrigerators. In fact, our body's natural mineral supply begins in the earth. Plants absorb minerals into their roots, passing them along to stems, leaves, and fruits. We then eat the mineral-rich plants or animals that have eaten the plants. Thus, corn on the cob and artichoke hearts are links in a conveyor belt that transports minerals from soil to human tissue.

Fruits, vegetables, whole grains, and milk provide the best supply of essential minerals, but, like vitamins, they are not found in adequate amounts in any single food. Even with a diet that appears well-balanced, you may still be

DIETERS, MONITOR VITAMIN INTAKE

Unlike fats, carbohydrates, and proteins, vitamins don't supply structure or energy to the body's tissues. Nevertheless, they are indispensable in cell maintenance, building, and energy-producing processes. Less than an adequate supply of one vitamin—a vitamin deficiency—sets off a chain reaction that impacts the formation of thousands of necessary chemical compounds.

Dieters, here's the point: A long-term, low-calorie diet could be negatively affecting your vitamin consumption. For example, with the standard, low-calorie diet meals available at the supermarket freezer, you could be getting 100% of your daily protein requirement and less than 25% of the daily requirements of certain essential vitamins. Be sure to check the labels—all the ingredients—if personally stylizing your diet. As a safeguard, take a multivitamin.

getting an inadequate supply. Taking a mineral tablet provides some insurance *if* the mineral tablet is properly constituted, but that's a big if. Some minerals must be in precise combinations to be absorbed by the body; some must be bound to other nutrients. And some, if taken alone, can cause physical problems, such as ulcers or diarrhea. Unfortunately, some tablet manufacturers don't concern themselves with these problems. It's best that you ask a pharmacist to help you select the best brand.

One mineral that has gotten a lot of attention in the past few years is calcium. Your mom was right when she insisted that you drink your milk! As mentioned in chapter 1, bones get stronger through weight training due to their pulling and tugging muscles during the activity. To help provide a strong foundation for your bones, eat a healthy diet with particular emphasis on calcium. If you're a calorie/cholesterol counter, you may be reluctant to add dairy foods. However, dairy foods provide 75% of the calcium in the U.S. food supply, and you can be selective about which sources to eat. Besides cheese, vitamin D-fortified lowfat and nonfat milk are good sources of vitamin D, which helps the body use calcium. These days yogurt comes in all flavors and mixes, from fat-free to low-fat to custardlike, fruit-filled creams. Also, foods such as broccoli, kale, and salmon with the bones are rich sources of calcium and better than a calcium supplement pill.

Minerals are as essential as vitamins to cell function. They participate in enzyme and hormone production, give structure to teeth and bones, and regulate muscle contractions and the conversion of food into energy. *All* cells need them to survive. Table 10.1 is a list of essential minerals.

TABLE 10.1 Essential Minerals

Needed in Large Amounts	Needed in Trace Amounts
Calcium	Iron
Potassium	Copper
Magnesium	Iodine
Sodium chloride	Fluoride
Phosphorus	Cobalt
Sulphur	Manganese
	Zinc
	Molybdenum
	Chromium
	Selenium

A deficiency of just one of the minerals will, in the least, wreck your work out. Before moving on, several minerals deserve special notice. They're the electrolytes.

The Electrolytes: Sodium, Potassium, Chloride

Every athlete has probably heard the term *electrolyte balance*. Electrolytes are mineral compounds that maintain a balance of body fluids, which is vital to the athlete's cooling system.

One electrolyte, sodium, is the blood's largest mineral constituent. Low salt level can lead to dehydration because the body needs salt to retain water. This is why generations of coaches have passed out salt tablets to their troops. They needn't do that, though, because the body's need for salt can be easily met with a normal diet. In fact, the average American's salt intake is 50 times greater than it need be! It's rare to find an American who isn't salty enough.

While too little salt causes dehydration, too much can lead to dehydration, too. How? Excess salt increases urination to rid the body of the excess. This increased urination drains fluid from the body, and the lack of fluid can overload the cooling system and lead to heat stroke.

Every time the body loses water, it loses potassium, which is vital to cellular function in the following, important way: During exercise, excess heat must be eliminated from the working muscles. Like all the body's internal heat, it is eliminated through the bloodstream. A discharge of potassium from muscle cells acts to widen the blood vessels, allowing more blood to reach and remove more heat. The immediate heat problem is solved, but a potassium problem is created. It won't be solved until more potassium is absorbed from the foods in the intestine.

Too little potassium produces that tired, run-down feeling you hear about in TV commercials, or the muscle cramps of dieting and training. Lucky for you, potassium is easily replaced with a glass of orange juice.

GETTING SPECIFIC: FDA DEFINITIONS OF SODIUM

Sodium free: less than 0.5 gram per serving

Low sodium: 140 milligrams or less per serving and, if the serving is 30 grams or less or 2 tablespoons or less, per 50 grams of the food

Very low sodium: 35 milligrams or less per serving and, if the serving is 30 grams or less or 2 tablespoons or less, per 50 grams of the food

Reduced or less sodium: at least 25% less per serving than reference food

Chloride is the last of the electrolytes, but, because it's less easily lost through dehydration, it is less likely to be responsible for a deficient state in the body. Like sodium, chloride comes to us in sufficient quantities through a normal diet. This broaches an important, concluding point: Do we need those expensive, heavily marketed sport drinks to replenish our electrolytes? Certainly not—like protein supplements, the sports drinks are more hype than help.

CLOSING SET

The weight trainer's diet is no different than the well-balanced diet of the average person except for an elevated intake of energy to meet the elevated energy expenditures attendant to training demands. The increased energy consumption should be provided through foods that conform to the well-balanced ratio of nutrients: 15% protein, 60% carbohydrates, and 25% fat. When energy needs are extreme—for example, during a competitive sports season or extensive cross training—the balance should be modified to reflect a higher percentage of carbohydrates and a lower percentage of fats and proteins.

Intense training, coupled with a well-balanced diet adequate to fulfill energy needs, will ensure success. It's that simple.

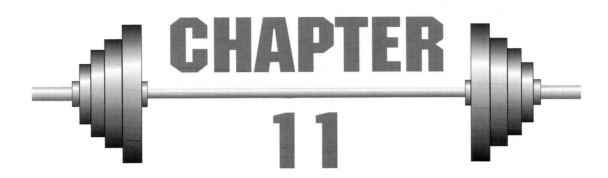

Weight Gain, Weight Loss

When dieters fight fat, their bodies fight back! In other words, your intellectualized goals might be contrary to your body's subliminal needs. Frustrated weight trainers have always suspected that such resistance is at work as pounds become increasingly harder to shed as the diet stretches into weeks and months. Those frustrated weight trainers are right.

That's the case for all other dieters too, whether couch potatoes or marathoners, fat or lean. The following sections outline some of the problems weight trained dieters face—whether the diet is designed to gain or lose weight.

THE BODY FEEDS ON ITSELF

Runner Jay Helgerson, a fellow who finished 52 marathons in 52 weeks, burned as many as 2,500 calories during a race or workout. He might burn another 2,200 just grocery shopping, taking out the garbage, and pressing the TV remote throughout the rest of the day. That's a total energy expenditure about 4,700 calories per day.

Some days, he consumed fewer calories than he burned, perhaps 500 fewer. Where did his body find that extra 500 calories of energy? His body dined on itself. That's right, there's a cannibal in all of us.

When the body runs short on food energy, it raids the biological pantry for stored fat and glycogen. Fat from fat cells and glycogen stored in the liver and muscle are easily converted into energy. The process has been refined through millions of years of evolutionary trials and errors. Modern weight-loss diet plans rely for success on this timeworn process of larger raids to drop body weight.

But the conditioned weight trainer is not your typical dieter. He or she may be at or near ideal body weight, so he or she doesn't want to follow the typical dieter's pattern. The weight trainer's emphasis is muscle. His or her goal is to *retain muscle* while losing a few pounds of fat. Meeting that goal requires careful attention to detail.

It is not uncommon to find a finely tuned weight trainer with as little as 2% body fat. What happens if that 2% of fat is entirely consumed by the body because the athlete hasn't been eating enough? After gobbling the available fat, the body satisfies its energy appetite with protein. Metaphorically, it feasts on protein that is part of that hard-earned muscle tissue. That's a serious problem for the weight trainer. The least that will happen is loss of muscle efficiency as he or she veers toward malnourishment.

The general recommendation from doctors and sports trainers is that the athlete and nonathlete alike keep a little body fat (about 10% of body weight) "hanging around" for food emergencies. The rationale is that it's safer to carry around a few excess, consumable pounds than to take the chance of burning muscle that has taken months or years to build. The average weight trainer, however, abhors excess fat, and if you fall into that category, play it healthy by meticulously monitoring your calorie intake, making sure to protect your gains with enough calories to meet your daily energy expenditures.

GAINING MUSCLE WHILE LOSING WEIGHT? IT WON'T HAPPEN

In the previous section, we explored the possibility of the weight trainer's body consuming its own muscle tissue as a last resource for energy. A corollary is: The weight trainer won't gain muscle tissue while on a weight-loss diet.

Intuition and advertising—the before and after pictures—tell us that we can gain muscle while losing weight, but that's not true. A negative energy balance, burning more calories than the food eaten provides, inhibits muscle growth. Why?

The body's genetic agenda is prioritized to maintain health and life at all costs. Consistent with this agenda, energy expenditures are prioritized when available energy is in short supply. Topping the list of energy dependent priorities is the basic metabolism that keeps the body alive, such as heartbeat and temperature control.

Next in line for an energy handout is tissue *maintenance*, keeping the status quo of physical structures. In other words, the body opts to protect the muscle tissue, carbohydrate storehouses, and fat cells present when the weight-loss, lower energy diet began. New tissue—this includes building more muscle tissue—is the last on the list of priorities when allocating scarce energy. The body uses energy to replenish those ugly fat cells and carbohydrate stores before adding any new muscle tissue.

What about those before-and-after pictures? Are they retouched? Not necessarily. Just dieting away the layer of subcutaneous fat that covers the muscle in the before picture creates a bigger, more impressive after picture.

There's another factor to consider: Muscle tissue previously built through weight training and lost when left dormant through a layoff or reduction in workout intensity will increase in volume, even during a diet. The renewed intensity merely triggers a "maintenance response," as if the tissue had never been lost. In fact, the basic strength-size structures (myofibrils) hadn't been lost.

Reinvigorating the size and strength of old muscle tissue is possible during a weight-loss diet; but don't count on *new* muscle tissue. It won't happen. Gaining new muscle requires the stress of weight training and a positive energy balance.

STRENGTH AND ENDURANCE DROP, TOO!

The first stages of a diet-exercise routine typically produce a new vitality. It seems that we're full of energy and gaining strength. Strength might, in fact, improve in the short term as neural adaptations augment the new efficiency of the new exercise routines. Don't be fooled, though: Chronic calorie restrictions impair both strength and muscular efficiency by decreasing the muscles' glycogen stores, and that sense of vitality will turn to lethargy over time with extreme calorie restrictions.

BULK UP, CUT DOWN

Bulking up is bodybuilding vernacular for adding both fat and muscle. The bodybuilder bulks up in the off-season, adding muscle to his frame. Conversely, he "cuts" the fat from his body before competition by dieting to remove the excess fat that covers the combination of newly developed and old muscle tissue. Can he stop this biological yo-yo effect, eating just enough to add muscle but not fat?

Practically speaking, no. Adding new muscle tissue requires a positive energy balance; that is, more energy consumption than needed to maintain existing tissue and energy-consuming activities. Here's the rub: The extra energy consumed is stored as fat. Hence, in practice, muscle growth leads to more fat. Why "in practice?" Because it's impractical to regulate caloric intake to precisely match expenditures (including new muscle tissue). A few calories too few will prevent muscle growth; a few too many will add fat. That doesn't mean that a gram of fat is stored with every gram of new muscle. As noted above, existing muscle can be retained while losing fat. It simply means, in practice, that new muscle tissue cannot be added without adding just a tiny globule of fat.

The bottom line: Extra food, supplying extra energy, is a requirement of muscle building. Some of that food will add muscle, if heavy training goes hand-in-hand with heavy eating. Some of that food piles on as fat, but that's

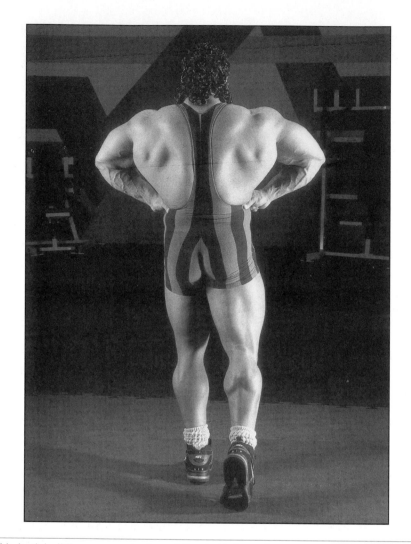

"Bulking up" is bodybuilding vernacular for adding both fat and muscle. As contest time approaches, the bodybuilder reduces caloric intake, selectively shedding the fat while retaining most of the added muscle.

no big deal—after adding 50 pounds of muscle and a few pounds of fat, the fat can be burned away to reveal the remarkable changes lying below.

SPOT REDUCING: IT'S IN THE EYE

Spot reducing—selectively losing fat at a particular body part through dieting—won't happen. During a weight-loss diet, the body operates as an equal opportunity depleter: The proportion of fat lost at the calves is the same as the proportion of fat lost at the waistline.

What about the spot-reduction of fat through exercise? That won't happen either. A thousand squats a day won't shed ugly fat from the hips. Any fat lost from the squats will be lost from the arms as readily as the hips.

Combining exercise and diet creates the *appearance* of spot reduction with little actual fat loss, especially after a layoff. For example, the weight trainer can "deflate" the girth of the stomach with just a little overall body fat reduction. He can "inflate" the existing muscles of the shoulders and chest through the resumption of intense training. The changed proportions from the slightly smaller stomach and slightly larger shoulders visually simulate spot reduction, when, in fact, body fat at shoulder and stomach are proportional to initial content.

A reiterated caveat: Muscle mass *can't be added* during a weight-loss diet. Existing muscle mass *can be maintained* during the diet as long as enough stored fats and consumed carbohydrates are available to meet the body's energy needs. Too little of each can stimulate the body to ravish your muscle's protein structures for the needed energy.

SELECTIVE MUSCLE LOSS

At the 1977 Mr. America Contest, Mae West said about Dave Johns, the winner: "He's got it all, and it's all in the right places." Which leads to an awkward segue: Could he have lost a little muscle from the wrong places if he chose?

Most weight trainers want to streamline because excess baggage slows movement, more quickly tires the body, or just plain looks bad. Official race-track handicappers have long used this fact to even their fields, adding weight to the stronger horses to slow them down. Poky nags are assigned less weight.

Muscle, too, can be excess baggage that adversely affects performance. For the bodybuilder, too much muscle in a particular spot might detract from overall symmetry. For the movement-dependent athlete, excess muscle mass is any muscle mass detracting from the power of a sport-specific movement.

How can you target a particular muscle for tissue loss? Easy: Don't overload it. Muscles shrink, or atrophy, from disuse. The bigger the muscle, the quicker it weakens and shrinks from lack of use. And shrunken muscles weigh less. If you discontinue overloading muscles not needed for sports success—if you're a soccer player and neglect your biceps, for example—the result is a selective loss of muscle mass.

GETTING BETTER, NOT JUST BIGGER

Gaining weight isn't rocket science: Stuff more Twinkies down the hatch than needed to satisfy energy demands and you'll gain weight. Gaining muscle, however, takes more effort than just raising a forkful of grits to your mouth—it takes hard training.

All excess calories are stored as fat, even those calories that pass the lips as the purest of proteins and carbohydrates. That presents a dilemma for athletes: They don't want weight for weight's sake; extra weight, if not involved muscle, slows movement. Weight per se doesn't add to any push, pull, twist, or turn needed for any sport. Imagine Andre Agassi competing in a tennis tournament with a 25-pound lead belt around his waist. Yet many athletes seek just such a handicap without realizing it. They seek more size without considering the consequences to movement.

Added body fat slows movements. Fat adversely affects the cardiovascular system, too. The heart and bloodstream have that much more tissue to supply with nutrients and oxygen. That extra heart action and blood supply could be much better used to feed working muscles.

A gain in muscular body weight through weight training might be desirable. Added muscle might mean faster, more powerful movements. Why qualify the foregoing statements with

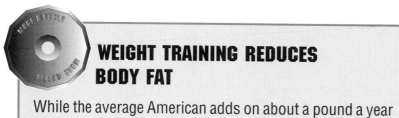

WEIGHT TRAINING REDUCES BODY FAT

While the average American adds on about a pound a year to his or her weight, people who strength train regularly have to eat 15% more calories in order to maintain their weight. As they weight train, they lose body fat; however, they make strength gains, increasing the amount of weight they could lift by 24% to 92%.

"might"? Because a positive effect depends on a selective increase. Add size and strength to muscles that significantly contribute to your event; don't add muscle that can diminish your speed. A 20-inch neck isn't going to help a bowler get more strikes. Mr. Universe-like biceps won't help a soccer player kick more goals. On the other hand, more muscular legs will probably help both.

If you're weight training to increase your athletic performance, consider the effect of unnecessary pounds, both fat and muscle. Add muscle mass only where that mass will power your athletic success.

CRASH WEIGHT LOSS: A HOMEOSTATIC SHOCK!

In the fall of 1980, heavyweight boxing champion Larry Holmes defended his title against aging ex-champ Muhammad Ali in Las Vegas. Holmes had little trouble, as Ali's trainer, Angelo Dundee, threw in the towel before the start of the 11th round.

Apart from the handicap of age, Ali was fighting the effects of crash weight loss. Two months before the fight he had weighed 256 pounds. By the official weigh-in he had gone down to 217 1/2. That's more than 38 pounds in 2 months. He lost fat. He lost muscle. He lost water. He lost homeostasis—an ongoing balance in all the body's systems.

Ali went too far. He restricted his carbohydrate intake to the point that his body fed on muscle tissue for energy needs. His unbalanced diet, with a concurrent change in physical activity, threw the body's metabolic processes into disarray. Reduced nutrients caused an enzyme imbalance. Energy was markedly out of balance. The assault on homeostatic tranquillity was exacerbated by Ali's consumption of a thyroid medication to increase water loss. The excess water loss produced dehydration, a water imbalance.

HEALTHY WEIGHT LOSS METHODS

Weight trainers wanting to lose weight in conjunction with a weight training program should follow the safe, accepted method of losing one to two pounds per week. That method requires a daily deficit of 500 to 1,000 calories through a combination of less food and increased physical activity.

In real terms, that's no more than skipping dessert (a small one at that) and taking an after dinner walk. That's all it takes to lose weight and stay healthy.

The lesson taken from Ali's ordeal is clear: Quick weight losses shock your body, which is used to a repetition of the same old things, its consistent habits. Consistent habits allow for internal consistency. A marked inconsistency shocks the system.

One such habit relates to diet, the eating pattern you've developed over the years. Your body has become accustomed to a rather consistent (or inconsistent) pattern of quantities and ingredients. A sudden change—such as missed meals—causes your insides to respond with cravings, headaches, or hunger pangs. The digestive system and absorption process don't mesh gears. It takes time for the body to adjust its assembly line to changes in quantity and ingredients.

Adaptations must occur all along the metabolic chain; from the change in tension of the muscle cells lining the digestive tract to the brain's relative share of blood glucose. That's why a moderate diet is less shocking to homeostasis (i.e., ongoing balance) than an extreme diet. It is also the reason why it's easier to slowly reduce coffee consumption than to go "cold turkey." The complexity of the metabolic chain is why big change takes time.

Losing weight safely and wisely takes time. Be patient, so that your body as a whole can cope with the changes. Think long term; a consistent, moderate approach to weight training and diet will give you the positive results you're after without the negative side effects of a crash diet. Rapid weight loss is usually due to the loss of water, which is dangerous.

Lose weight the sensible, recommended way, not the Ali way. Be content with a one to two pound loss per week—a loss that can be achieved with a daily 500- to 1,000-calorie deficit. That way, you'll not find yourself out on your feet, holding on for dear life.

One final note on this: Protein requirements increase when the diet provides fewer calories than the body expends, because the body's energy expenditures must be met before the body can synthesize protein. Hence, if you're on a restricted calorie diet, you should be sure to eat more protein. The extra calories accompanying the extra protein can be compensated through a further reduction in calories from fat.

CLOSING SET

Patience is the key to safe weight gain and weight loss. Crash diets or crash weight-gain diets don't work over the long haul, with or without weight training. A crash or fad diet is apt to lead to malnourishment and lethargy.

The key to successful dieting is orchestrating and following a plan that incrementally changes diet and exercise routines. Starving or stuffing "shocks" the body into a defensive mode. Slowly coax your body to adapt to changes in consumption, and it will be less likely to fight back with a salvo of painful defenses.

When restricting energy consumption by restricting intake, closely monitor your intake of protein, carbohydrates, vitamins, and minerals to assure that you meet your basic needs. You won't gain muscle—but you can maintain muscle—on a calorie deficit diet. In practice, a calorie deficit diet is likely to adversely affect your strength and muscular endurance.

Above all, respect the recommendation that your energy deficit run no greater than 500 to 1,000 calories per day, resulting from a combination of calorie reduction and increased physical activity.

CHAPTER 12

Training Safely and Nursing Injuries

All athletes subject their bodies to extraordinary stresses that can lead to an assortment of injuries. As you would suspect, weight training injuries most often involve muscles. Although most weight room injuries are minor—soreness is the usual culprit—no injury should be treated as routine. Every injury should be considered something of an emergency, calling for immediate attention and evaluation. Serious muscle injuries—strains, sprains, and tears—are rare. A broken bone is an extraordinary rarity, smashed toes less so. But those that do occur can usually be traced to faulty technique, lack of supervision, an unnecessarily large overload, or inattentiveness.

An injury requires accurate diagnosis and treatment, which requires the intervention of a trained professional. Self-treatment through self-help books and self-diagnosis should be discarded as a matter of policy. Don't self-treat: Combine your input with the knowledge of a trained professional to effect an appropriate treatment plan.

Many of the sections in this chapter include generally accepted methods of emergency treatment. Whether self-administered or performed by a trainer, coach, or doctor, the procedures are applicable to the usual athletic injuries. There are some healthy doses of preventive medicine prescribed here, too, beginning with generally recognized safety procedures.

RULES FOR SAFE TRAINING

Although infrequent, the possibility of injury is present every time a weight trainer enters the weight room. The following accepted safety guidelines will reduce that possibility.

Correct technique: Learn to do it right! As a rule of thumb, ballistic movements—jerks and bounces—are inappropriate for most exercises, whether performed with free weights or machines. Additional technical advice can be gleaned from the exercise descriptions in this book or from the advice of an experienced supervisor.

Breathing during exercise: Breathe naturally when lifting weights. Don't intentionally hold your breath: Intrathoracic blood pressure rises during the lift through a combination of muscular contractions and the intentionally inflated lungs. Further fallout from holding the breath is the restriction of venous blood flow returning to the heart, leading to lower heart volume and decreased blood flow to the brain. As a general guideline, exhale during the lifting movement (the effort phase) and inhale during the lowering movement (the rest phase).

Shoes: Make sure they're tied and can withstand lateral motion: Running shoes are usually inadequate for the stresses of weight training. Basketball shoes work great. Worn heels can lead to a sprained ankle or worse.

Supervision: Especially for beginners, nothing replaces an experienced supervisor who can recognize potential problems before they lead to injury.

Spotters: The rule of thumb: Work with a spotter with the knowledge and capacity to help in an emergency—during a bench press, squat, or any other lift during which the lifter can get "stuck" under a weight.

Free weights: When exercising with free weights, it's important to check the following, often overlooked factors:

- ◆ Collars prevent plates from sliding from the ends of bars, smashing toes, or leaving the lifter with a precariously unbalanced bar. Lifting without collars is *the number one cause of weight room injuries.*

- ◆ Maintain a balanced load throughout the loading process. Pay particular attention when adding plates to a bar supported on a rack (e.g., bench press or squat rack). A heavy side can cause the bar to tilt and come crashing down.

- ◆ Take care that you have enough room to complete your lift. This is of the utmost importance when exercising in a crowded gym. Just like while driving a car, you must be on the lookout for the other person.

- ◆ Before each set, make sure the plates are tight against the stops and the collars snug against plates. A few inches of plate displacement on one end of the bar decreases balance while increasing the probability of an accident.

- ◆ Don't drop the barbells or dumbbells. Control the free weight throughout the exercise movement. Massive objects and gravity combine for obvious safety hazards. Furthermore, you'll wear out your welcome in the gym.

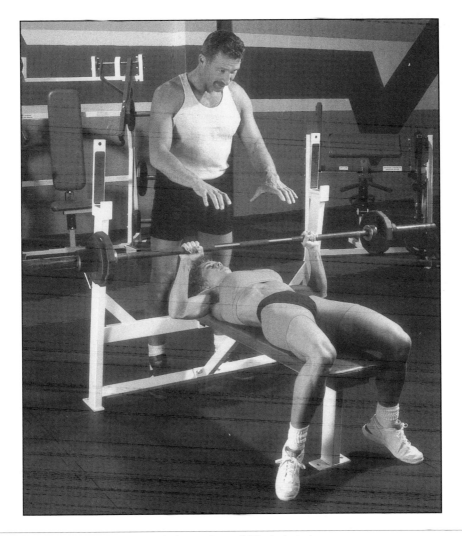

Work with a spotter who has the knowledge and capability to help in an emergency.

Machines: The machine must fit *your* body to be both safe and effective as a training vehicle. The typical weight training machine doesn't fit all body sizes; it's manufactured to meet average needs. Very large or very small bodies can be endangered if forced to contort to the machine's size or range of motion. If the machine doesn't fit, duplicate the motion with a free weight. There are ongoing safety checks, too:

◆ The same caveats for free weights apply to machines: control the momentum of the exercise movement; no bounces and no jerks.

◆ Check frayed cables, worn belts, loose pads, weight-stack pins, and seat locks before each set.

◆ Stay clear of moving parts—including the weight stack—when another person is using the machine. Never place your hands between weight stacks!

◆ When new to the machine, have an experienced user teach you the proper form, including correct entry and exit. Check the manufacturer's placard, too, for specific instructions!

Warm-up: The primary objective of a warm-up is injury prevention. Select a group of warm-up exercises that incorporate all major muscle groups. Warm-up exercises raise body temperatures, increasing the rate of muscle metabolism, resulting *in increased speed of contraction.* The muscles are then ready for the more intense exercise movements that follow.

Stretch: Like the warm-up, stretching prepares the muscles and joints for more intense exercise movements. The stretching relaxes the muscle fibers, allowing for a greater range of motion in the joint. Consequently, there is a lesser chance of injury from the extended motion of the exercise movement. Most trainers recommend stretching before and after the exercise session.

Sharp pain during exercise: An extreme, sharp pain—a different effect than common muscular soreness—is a signal to *stop training immediately!* Assess the problem before resuming training.

EMERGENCY TREATMENT: REST, ICE, COMPRESSION, ELEVATION

R.I.C.E. is an acronym for the emergency treatment of injuries—Rest, Ice, Compression, and Elevation. It may be timeworn, but it's still good general advice. Here it is in full form.

◆ **R**est: Rest at the first sign of injury. In other words, stop training!
◆ **I**ce: Immediately apply ice to limit swelling.
◆ **C**ompression: Apply pressure to the injured area to limit swelling.
◆ **E**levation: Raise the injury above the heart, reducing blood pressure to the injured area.

If not *R.I.C.E.*, a biography of a trainer's life might aptly be titled *The Iceman Cureth*. Trainers probably use more ice than bartenders. That's because applying an icebag or other cold compress to an injured area of the body reduces swelling in all kinds of injuries. The application of cold constricts, or narrows, the broken blood vessels. That means less bleeding into the healthy tissue, and less bleeding leads to less swelling and less pain.

Cold should be applied in cycles of 30 minutes on and 30 minutes off throughout the two-day period following a muscle injury. You're probably not going to have the stamina or patience to do it around the clock, or the discomfort tolerance to endure applications lasting longer than 30 minutes, but do try to do as many as 30-minute cycles as you can. The more frequently you apply the cold, the shorter and less severe the internal bleeding.

It's best to use a commercial icebag or ice cubes wrapped in a towel. The surface of the bag or towel acts as a safety buffer. Don't apply freezing ice directly to your warm skin. You don't need frostbite added to your troubles.

Along with applying enough ice to the injured area to make it feel like a penguin's wing, wrap it with an elastic bandage. Again, the reason is to reduce swelling from the broken blood vessels in the injured muscle tissue. The compression from the bandage won't permit blood to seep into surrounding tissue. The wrap should be applied tightly enough to block normal circulation. If a bone break is suspected, the wrap should be replaced by a splint, if possible, until professional medical help arrives.

Raising the injured part above the level of the heart will slow the seepage of blood from the damaged vessels. Of course, not all injuries are located such that this advice can be followed, but when possible elevate the injury while applying cold and a compression wrap. Every little bit helps to stop the damaging swelling.

Ice should be applied from 24 to 72 hours to be safe. If there's a lot of swelling after 72 hours, ice should be continued. Heat should not be applied until swelling is reduced. After 24 to 72 hours of ice, the weight trainer is probably ready to move from the Arctic to the tropics, so to speak. The blood vessels have probably mended enough to stop additional seepage, and the heat will increase circulation, which in turn will deliver more of the blood's healing agents to the injury. Most doctors and trainers recommend heating the injured area throughout the recuperative period.

Heat is useful for virtually any type of athletic injury and can be delivered in many ways. The precise method is decided by the depth of the injury. A near-surface bruise can be treated with surface applications: perhaps hot towels, hydroculators (small, simple, portable devices that retain heat), heating pads, or heat lamps.

If a bruised, strained, or torn muscle happens to be deep within the limb or thorax (that part of the trunk between the neck and abdomen), the surface application of heat won't reach the injured tissue. Thus, it's necessary to use a more sophisticated device, an ultrasonic vibrator, which produces hundreds of thousands of sound vibrations per minute. These vibrations heat the deep tissue. Most training rooms have one, or see your medical doctor and physical therapist about its use.

COMMON (AND UNCOMMON) MUSCLE INJURIES

Anything can happen during a workout: The ceiling could collapse on an unsuspecting soul during a set of curls—that literally happened at the original Gold's Gym. Of course, there are more predictable injuries. Those, as you probably suspect, involve muscle. A look at the most common muscle injuries, along with some precautions and treatment advice, follows.

Myositis: Sore Muscles

Al Bundy, in the television series "Married With Children," avoids exercise. He squats to fit a pair of shoes on a customer's foot and walks to the refrigerator several times a day. Uncharacteristically, he spends Sunday afternoon playing softball with his wife's family at a picnic outing. A pleasant day concludes with a highly-piled plate of fried chicken and potato salad. The next morning, as he rolls out of bed, is anything but pleasant. He's suffering from myositis, also referred to as delayed onset muscle soreness.

Myositis is not a dread disease spread by bacteria from rotting toadstools; it is merely the fancy name for muscle soreness—that common pain most people wake up with the day after being a once-a-year left halfback. *It is generalized,* low-level, omnipresent soreness of overused muscles. *It is not spot-specific,* the characteristic of pain that stems from a distinct location of a muscle tear or rupture.

What is the physiological basis for the pain? If Bundy could peel back the skin and examine his tender muscle tissue with a microscope, he would find it inflamed and mildly swollen. Closer examination would find cell membranes torn. Cellular material would be leaking through the tears. White blood cells would be coursing through the damaged tissue. If his muscle cells had vocal chords, he'd hear a chorus of moans with each contraction.

Unlike strains and ruptures, the effects of myositis disappear more quickly if mild exercise is continued. Apparently, the increased circulation helps induce healing. There have been anecdotal reports that soaking in a hot tub comforts those sore, aching muscles, too.

Muscle Cramps: An Extended Contraction

A long, intense workout can be an arduous affair, repeatedly pushing the muscle to overload tension, draining energy stores, taxing recovery mechanisms. It's not uncommon for a muscle to cramp during or after an all-out workout.

A muscle cramp (or charley horse or spasm) is a muscle contraction that lasts too long—a muscle that won't *un*-contract. Cramps can result from electrolyte (i.e., sodium, potassium, chloride, magnesium) depletion, usually in conjunction with dehydration. Diagnosis is usually no problem, because a cramp is easily recognizable as a painful, unexpected tightening of the muscle. They're most common in the hamstrings, calves, and feet. The cramp may form a "lump" and it always hurts.

Since a cramp is a prolonged contraction—sometimes accompanied by a minor tear—the immediate treatment is to relax the muscle. That's accomplished by stretching the muscle to its normal, relaxed position. For example, a cramped calf can be relaxed by pulling the toes toward the shin, stretching the contracting muscle into submission. After stretching, massaging the cramped muscle usually helps. Massage is simply a variation of relaxing the muscle through stretching. As the muscle is manipulated and stretched by the fingers, the contracting fibers relax.

The muscle can be used, with caution, immediately after the cramp subsides. Caution is called for because the cramp may be indicative of a slight muscle tear, and a slight muscle tear can become severe if the injured muscle is subjected to continued demands.

If chronic cramps are a problem, a little preventive stretching before exercise might be a solution. Stretch those troublesome muscle groups at least once a day.

Muscle Strain: Partially Torn Muscle

It is common in training rooms to hear talk—or moans—about a pulled hamstring or a pulled groin muscle. A muscle pull is the same thing as a muscle strain: a partial tear across the width of the muscle. The damaged muscle, like a similarly torn rubber band or rope, still works, but with less strength—the train of force is broken at the tear.

From a surface examination, it's hard to distinguish a strained muscle from other muscle injuries described in this section. As in some of the other injuries beneath the skin's surface, at the point of the tear, the muscle is bleeding, resulting in surface swelling and lots of pain.

Even when a strain is correctly diagnosed, trainers and doctors have difficulty determining its degree of seriousness. The tear may be small or large, involving only a few fibers or the greater part of the muscle's width.

Treat a suspected muscle strain with R.I.C.E. Don't stress the muscle for several days. Even then, be cautious when returning to the weight room. Better to miss a few workouts than risk a more serious tear.

Muscle Rupture: A Complete Tear

A ruptured muscle is analogous to an extended rubber band, which, when cut, recoils in two different directions. It is usually caused by a sudden, gross overload. Fortunately, a muscle rupture is much less common in sports than a muscle strain or partial tear. Among weight lifters, ruptured biceps and pectorals are the most common forms of this generally uncommon injury.

There's no doubt when a rupture occurs. The severed halves, unable to generate movement, recoil toward the bones to which they are attached. The injury produces extreme pain and swelling; the internal bleeding is greater than with a strain, because more muscle tissue is torn.

Sometimes a ruptured muscle is misdiagnosed as a ruptured tendon, since both put a joint or limb out of commission. Most sports doctors can distinguish the difference by the location of greatest pain. If the injury is to a tendon, the pain will be closer to the tendon's insertion at the bone. If it's a ruptured muscle, the worst pain will be somewhere along its "belly" (i.e., the middle of the muscle, which is usually also its thickest part).

Again, R.I.C.E. is the immediate prescription. It won't mend anything, but it will inhibit swelling, and that, in turn, will help diminish the pain. The only possible cure is a surgical procedure to sew the severed ends together again.

The longer the muscle is left damaged, the more atrophy will inhibit recovery, so prompt medical treatment is essential.

A positive note is that all is not lost when an athlete ruptures a muscle. Surgery often leads to full recovery and renewed use.

Scar Tissue: Mother Nature's Stitches

Scar tissue is nature's needle and thread, stitching together torn tissue. Unfortunately, scar tissue can be a problem, causing persistent pain and a loss of flexibility near an old injury. How? Each time the muscle contracts, the healthy muscle tissue must overstretch to compensate for the relative understretch of the scar tissue.

The muscle is vulnerable to more tears or ruptures near the scar tissue. It's a vicious circle—tears develop scar tissue, which brings on more tears. Overcoming the scar-tissue conundrum requires improving the muscle's overall flexibility without heightening the possibility for additional injury. Common sense matches accepted medical advice in this case: Begin with mild stretching, *gradually* increasing the range of motion through subsequent workouts. Start easy and progress; don't start fast and regress.

LONG-TERM MAINTENANCE STRATEGIES

Diet and rest are two controllable factors in the weight trainer's repertoire that play an important role in body maintenance and injury prevention.

Without adequate nutrition and rest, muscles are more likely to fail under stress. Reactions and attention, dulled by lack of sleep, may fail in the clutch. Conversely, weight trainers who do fuel their bodies intelligently and are habitual with patterns of adequate rest not only enhance the rate of improvement, but will also lower their chances of getting hurt.

Not every injury can be avoided any more than every forest fire can be prevented, but the tips on conduct outside the gym will help your chances of remaining injury-free. They require little extra effort, so why not try them?

Diet

The previous two chapters in *More Muscle* have been devoted to food—what to eat, under what circumstances, and why. However, it's also worth noting diet's relationship to injury prevention.

The body manufactures thousands of different chemical compounds from the two dozen essential nutrients we get in the food we eat. Missing just one of these nutrients through improper food selection starts a chain reaction that limits production of hundreds of these needed compounds.

An easy example is a diet lacking potassium, a nutrient we lose every time we sweat. A potassium deficiency leads to a shortage of compounds that directly impact muscular strength, muscular endurance, and cardiovascular endurance. The bottom line: Usual demands on undernourished muscles can produce an injury.

An overload—the stimulus for improved performance—is impossible with an undernourished muscle.

Sleep and Rest

Weight training places extreme physical demands on bones, muscles, tendons, and joints. Picture a weight trainer overloading his body, set after overload set. Can his body perform to maximum capacity—maximum overload—if his body is tired or sleepy? Of course not.

Frogs and salamanders don't need to sleep, but human beings do. For a long time, scientists believed that sleep was the time when the body replaced worn-out cells and repaired damaged tissues. That has turned out not to be true—just as much repair work goes on during waking periods. The brain doesn't take time off, either; free from directing the body's walking, sitting, eating, and other activities, it dreams and carries on life-support activities!

Most researchers divide sleep into four stages. Stage one is a sort of twilight zone in which the person has no directed thoughts. In stage two the brain becomes more active and there is some dreaming. In stage three the body (here's the important point) is now totally relaxed; pulse and temperature are down. In stage four the person is in delta sleep, the deepest phase. People don't just sink into stage four and stay there until awakening; each stage is entered and exited several times a night.

More to the point, no two weight trainers have the same sleep needs. The customary eight hours is average, but each of us has to find what is best for him or her. Too little sleep will cause irritability and erratic reaction time, opening the door to a multitude of misjudgments and missteps that would easily be avoided by a well-rested athlete whose timing was "on."

Rest isn't limited to sleep. The muscles need rest periods—time off from physical activity—between training sessions. Overtraining (see page 11) results if the body hasn't had time to recuperate before subjecting it to another round of demands. Overtraining can lead to serious physical and psychological problems that the athlete could easily avoid with a little more rest.

The point to remember is that sleep and rest intervals between training sessions are as important to your training success as time in the gym.

RETURNING AFTER A LAYOFF

Detraining, a loss in strength or endurance, happens during a layoff. Hence, it makes sense to calculate the efficiency loss when returning to the gym. Don't expect to use the same weights, reps, and sets.

Detraining brings real physical change. The muscle cell shrinks, losing the support systems necessary for maximal contractions. The bones, tendons, and nervous system also are comparatively less active than what they were during peak training.

Some practical tips will help you safely return from an extended layoff. First, get your doctor's okay. Once in the weight room, higher than pre-layoff reps with fewer sets and lower weights are the menu for the first four weeks back, even if your enthusiasm is at a higher level. Thereafter, gradually increase the overload, bringing yourself to pre-layoff performance. In essence, it's like starting to train all over again.

Caution is a virtue when returning from a layoff. Maximum overload is an extreme jump in the demands placed on the muscles when compared to the lethargy of the layoff. Extreme soreness is a certainty, and worse—tears, strains, and ruptures—could easily happen. Take it easy.

CLOSING SET

Enter the weight room with safety as a top priority. Even before the weight room, take care that your diet and rest habits are commensurate with your weight training expectations and goals.

If you are injured, follow the emergency guidelines of rest, ice, compression, and elevation (R.I.C.E.). All injuries should be treated as emergencies. Take appropriate precautions before resuming training. Play it safe by seeking immediate, professional help for diagnosis and treatment of anything more than the most minor of injuries. Respond to any pain by immediately stopping training. Seek medical attention. It's better to be safe than sidelined.

Good luck, and have a safe, effective workout.

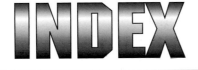

ABOUT THE AUTHOR

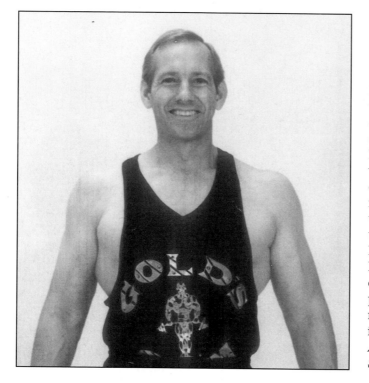

Ken Sprague is a pioneer and a giant in the fitness industry. He owned and operated the original Gold's Gym in Venice Beach, California, for more than a decade. Under his leadership, the gym grew from a small business that grossed less than $20,000 a year to a world-famous, multimillion-dollar conglomerate of fitness-related businesses and entertainment events with more than 400 locations worldwide. Because of this great success, Ken has been featured in hundreds of magazine and newspaper articles as well as on many television shows, including *60 Minutes*, *Good Morning America*, and *The Regis Philbin Show*.

Ken has 35 years of practical weight training experience as well as a Phi Beta Kappa science degree from the University of Oregon and advanced training in sports physiology and psychology. During his career, he has used his expertise to train dozens of world and national weight lifting and bodybuilding champions. He has also shared his knowledge by lecturing on weight training and by writing several books on the subject. *The Gold's Gym Book of Weight Training*, Ken's first book, raised the public's interest in working out with weights and was a catalyst for the fitness boom of the 1970s and 80s. His other books include *The Gold's Gym Book of Strength Training for Athletes*, *The Gold's Gym Book of Bodybuilding*, *The Athlete's Body*, *Sports Strength*, and *Weight and Strength Training for Kids and Teenagers*.

As an organizer of weight training and bodybuilding events, Ken has also been very successful. During his years at Gold's Gym, he directed national and international bodybuilding championships, Mr. America competitions, national power lifting championships, and the first women's bodybuilding exhibition. Today, Ken continues to write, teach, coach, and lecture about weight training. In his leisure time, he enjoys doing carpentry, taking fossil hunting field trips, and cross-training with his wife, Donna, and their son, Chris.